Beverly;

Thanks so much for your interest about my book and my writing!

Be free to call to chat?

Donna

MENOPAUSE or LUNACY
...*That* is the Question

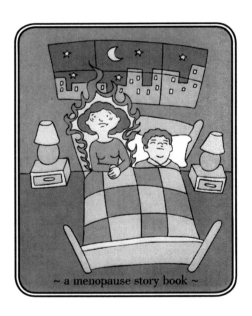

~ a menopause story book ~

DONNA FAYE RANDALL

Copyright © 2013 Donna Faye Randall.

All rights reserved. No part of this book may be used or reproduced by any means, graphic, electronic, or mechanical, including photocopying, recording, taping or by any information storage retrieval system without the written permission of the publisher except in the case of brief quotations embodied in critical articles and reviews.

Balboa Press books may be ordered through booksellers or by contacting:

Balboa Press
A Division of Hay House
1663 Liberty Drive
Bloomington, IN 47403
www.balboapress.com
1-(877) 407-4847

Because of the dynamic nature of the Internet, any web addresses or links contained in this book may have changed since publication and may no longer be valid. The views expressed in this work are solely those of the author and do not necessarily reflect the views of the publisher, and the publisher hereby disclaims any responsibility for them.

The author of this book does not dispense medical advice or prescribe the use of any technique as a form of treatment for physical, emotional, or medical problems without the advice of a physician, either directly or indirectly. The intent of the author is only to offer information of a general nature to help you in your quest for emotional and spiritual well-being. In the event you use any of the information in this book for yourself, which is your constitutional right, the author and the publisher assume no responsibility for your actions.

Any people depicted in stock imagery provided by Thinkstock are models, and such images are being used for illustrative purposes only.
Certain stock imagery © Thinkstock.

Printed in the United States of America.

ISBN: 978-1-4525-8169-9 (sc)
ISBN: 978-1-4525-8171-2 (hc)
ISBN: 978-1-4525-8170-5 (e)

Library of Congress Control Number: 2013916346

Balboa Press rev. date: 11/14/2013

Table of Contents

Can't Start at the Beginning—The Foreword xv

Acknowledgements xxi

Feeling Up, Feeling Down 1
    Daily Thoughts of a Menopausal Maniac—A Poem 3
    A Particularly Bad Morning 4
    The Chairs are NOT the Issue 8
    Watch Out for Your Job... and for Your
        Self-Esteem 13
    Menopause Killed the Cat—Almost 17
    Fighting the "Has-Been" Feeling 24
    It Can't be Getting Worse, Can it? 27

A Mind Blowing Experience 37
    Confessions of a Formerly Organized Woman 39
    Am I Budgeting-Inept or Is This Menopause? 43
    Menopause—The Perfect Time to Work on
        Your Own...From Home 47
    Rex Forgotten 51

In Search of a Brain—Ideally Mine 56
A Change in Perspective about a Dear Old Friend 60

I'll Never Look Like THAT! 71
Don't Call Me Ma'am 73
Always Wear a Pretty Camisole 78
A Sleeping Disorder called Menopause 82
From Zero to Full Time Menstruation, and
    Back Again 86
Hot Flashes—Yes? No? Can't Remember? 93
Did I Happen to Mention the Change in
    Body Shape? 99
Lotions, Potions, Serums, and a Good
    Deodorant 104
Going Off HRT—Easy Does it! 109
It's Unanimous about Menopause, Boating,
    and (Not) Sleeping! 115
The Road Back to Fitness 119

Finding Myself 129
Is it Possible to Forget This Stage? 131
Belly Dance—an Answer is Found 135
The Woman I'm Becoming and the Electric
    Pink Shoes 140
Life's a Blast! 143
The Hair's the Thing 148
Patient Times to Come 152
The New, Period Free, and Mostly Happy ME! ... 156

The Bottom Line?—The Afterword 165

Oh, Something More 169

Old Women (and Me)—A Poem 171

DEDICATED TO…

My Life-long Inspiration

For my mother, Katherine Leopoldine Nickel Randall

~ for teaching me, by example, to
be kind, fair, and caring

to all creatures great and small

~ and perhaps most of all, for passing along to me

her knowledge of how to appreciate

each and every

beautiful and distinctive sunset!

About the Relationship between Menopause and Lunacy

Many of the problems associated with menopause can be attributed to the undeniable overlapping of myth and medicine. A great deal can be understood regarding the type of myths attributed to female reproduction and its cessation when examining the societal shift from the matriarchal to the patriarchal. This shift affected how menopause was viewed both in society and medicine. It also affected the subsequent terminology used to describe the menopausal process and treatments developed to "correct" it.

A woman's bleeding was once considered a powerful cosmic event connected to the lunar cycles and the tides. This connection to the moon's cycle was later distorted and the connection between the wisdom of women and the tides denigrated. The word "lunacy" is the result of this denigration.

Excerpted with thanks from *Menopause Mayhem*, by Marleen M. Quint, Women's Health Advocate, from www.wildcelt.com *Women's Health Forum*.

With Thanks to...

Billy Joel,
in his song entitled *You May be Right*,
for the reminder that craziness
isn't necessarily negative:

You may be right
I may be crazy
But it just might be a lunatic you're looking for
(songmeanings.com)

and to

Mark Knopfler & Emmylou Harris
in the song entitled *Belle Start*,
for their inspiration to put writing
ahead of a full-time income:

You can't play it safe
and still go down in history
(decoda.com)

Can't Start at the Beginning— The Foreword

To write about menopause in a linear fashion, including attempting to start at the beginning, would do the entire topic injustice. You see, the menopause experience simply isn't linear.

First of all, it seems most of us don't know we are in menopause (unless it is prompted surgically) until well after we are into it and have become completely convinced that we are becoming lunatics. Well, at least that was my experience, perhaps accentuated by my somewhat earlier-than-usual onset of menopause. So when I started to go crazy, it didn't even occur to me (a former sexuality educator) that menopause was an option as the reason why. And based on my own experience, and that of many other women with whom I've spoken, I think it safe to say that the going-crazy process is gradual, so you really don't notice it happening—except that you are all stressed out—until something or someone helps you figure it out.

In my case, that something was a series of events and that someone was a Mz. Lezlee, a fairly new, but close, girlfriend—a woman I came to know through a former place of employment, where I also encountered Philippe, my man. I met them both for very good reasons, not the least of which was to help me through menopause. Meeting Philippe has proved to be beneficial on many fronts, and I digress often to this Philippe, who is helping me to age gracefully—a nice departure from desperately clinging to my youth.

Now, getting back to the subject of menopause—the true subject of this book—I clearly remember when Mz. Lezlee identified my menopausal state. Lezlee and I had known each other for a year and a bit, I think. Now wait a minute. It seems I can't clearly remember when my buddy identified me as a woman going through "the change of life". Well, of course I can't remember the chronology of it all! I generally can't remember if I paid my bills, or if I paid said bills to the appropriate company, much less remember exactly when any one event occurred in my life. But, bear with me. I will tell you how I first learned that I had a good excuse for my craziness, even though I can't tell you exactly when—except that I've obviously had that good excuse for some time. Although I can't quite remember the events leading up to this particular day, I know they had something to do with me fussing about my growing relationship with Philippe. In the course of one day, I'd sent four emails to Mz. Lezlee, with each one describing a complete reversal of my emotional state from that of the previous message. In other words, I was up and down like a yo-yo all day. I had just hit the "send" button to pass along message number four, when my phone rang. When I answered the phone, the voice of Mz. Lezlee quickly enquired, "You do know what's happening to you, don't you?" When I confessed that yes, I did know that I was going *$&#%* crazy, my kind friend replied, "Yes you are, but there is a perfectly good reason for it: you, dear girlfriend, are menopausal."

Well, you could have heard a pin drop as my poor, little brain desperately tried to process this new piece of information. How could I be in menopause when I was only 46 years old? Yes, of course, my periods had been extremely wacky, but they'd been wacky off and on since my tubal ligation back in 1995, I think it was—or maybe it was 1994. Who knows? (Or as my very good friend, dear Joy, would say, "Whose nose?". You see, Joy is very clever and cute with words. Or at least she was, back there and then, quite likely because neither of us was menopausal, so she still had the brainpower to be clever and I still had the brainpower to understand said cleverness.)

Could it really be true that these horrific emotional swings I'd been experiencing, more and more over the past few years, might be blamed on something other than the onset of lunacy? When did it begin? What influence had it had on my ability to make good decisions in my life? Was this why I was so tired and hardly able to do my job, let alone accomplish much else?

I was at once elated, concerned, and confused about what this news meant and where it would take me. But if you'll stick with me, I'll attempt to figure it all out while sharing my thoughts, feelings, and investigations with you, in the hope of passing along insights into the rigors and joys of this usually belittled, sometimes ignored, and almost always misunderstood stage of a woman's life. But remember; don't expect my accounts to be provided in a linear fashion!

As a woman-of-a-certain-age in the throes of menopause, who has a pretty good sense of humor, I offer you this book as an adjunct to the more serious and factual books written on the same topic—books you might already have read, might read in the future, or might never read. I've found in my life that just a spoonful of humor helps us endure even the more trying of life's experiences. The ability to laugh at oneself is a priceless gift and I'm excited to give you an insight into the menopausal experience in a way that will make or help you chuckle, or perhaps even guffaw with great glee, and experience at least a few deep and delicious belly laughs. Whether you've been there and done that—are there and doing that—think you are going crazy and can't figure out why—know you will one day be there and doing that—or know and love someone who is acting crazy and might be there and doing that—this is book is for you—honest! And knowing that almost everyone everywhere is leading a busy life, I've chosen to keep the book short and divide it into little anecdotes, herein called scenarios. They are designed to provide nuggets of information in a nutshell. You can read them in any order, and possibly time and time again, and pretty much anywhere. And, they just might help you pass the time while you wait, once again, for a woman-of-a-certain-age, because she can't find her car keys or doesn't remember making a lunch date with you because she has misplaced her daybook so doesn't know what day it is. I hope you will enjoy your read, laugh often, and learn lots. Mostly, I hope to help you answer the question posed in the title of this book, which quite likely is a resounding "yes"—yes, you or your loved one might well be experiencing both menopause and lunacy!

Acknowledgements

In the beginning—
my parents and brothers for my love of language, slightly twisted sense of humor, and my tendency to observe and question everything.

Throughout school—
my teachers and mentors from Grade 1 through to my doctoral studies for encouraging me to keep writing and helping me hone my skills, and DMG who called me a writer way back when.

During the journey called menopause—
my girlfriend for identifying my menopause and therefore my lunacy; my man for his patience, comfort, and good humor; and loads of female commiserations.

Through the book conception, writing, and production process—
everyone who listened to me blather on about each idea at every phase of this very long process, including lots

of women with whom I discussed my book, who loved the idea, and wanted to read it *now*.

And, last but not least—
the readers who took the time and made the effort to provide concrete recommendations (you know who you are); *my* editor, Mary Guilfoyle, who appeared serendipitously, got it, and worked closely with me to improve the product while getting it done; *my* web site designer, Sarah Donaldson, for helping define (refine?) my persona; and the team at Balboa Press, who helped pull it all together.

Feeling Up, Feeling Down

The emotional changes and
challenges of menopause

Daily Thoughts of a Menopausal Maniac—A Poem

~ inspired by P. K. Page and Anny Scoones
… along with Mable and Matilda,
the Gloucester Old Spots of Glamorgan ~

Oh my, oh my,
I forlornly cry!
Just tell me why
I must toil so
to get through each day
when so often
I just want to die.

With Glee, I see
in front of me
the bliss with which we
live each day …
in perfect harmony.

These ups and downs
and grins and frowns
reveal I'm out of control;
but now I see,
they are part of me …
this truly pathetic soul.

Donna Faye Randall

A Particularly Bad Morning

Many people say I'm not a morning person, but I correct them and say that I like mornings, as long as they don't start too early and I can ease into them. For example, I love to see the sunshine through the hatch of my partner's and my sailboat, while I snuggle with him under the covers of our bed in the V-berth (the pointy end of the boat).

As part of this journey called menopause, mornings have taken on new twists for me—one of which I'm not particularly fond. Because of hot flashes, often I don't sleep well. Of late, I've taken to awakening at about 5am, one and a half hours before my alarm rings on weekdays. Usually, I'm awake for a wee while before I realize it, and then once I do realize I'm awake, my brain decides to focus on things particularly disturbing or stressful (or, on those special mornings, both), and I don't return to sleep until about one half hour before my alarm rings. Of course, I then feel absolutely dreadful upon hearing the alarm, knowing I've started yet another day feeling like death warmed-over (to quote my dearly departed father).

This morning was one of those dreadful mornings. Not only did my brain focus on things particularly disturbing and stressful, but also I found myself crying as a result. I rose to cry in the bathroom so I would not awaken the love o' my life who was spending the night with me, and to blow my nose so I could breathe again. While I was partially successful with the breathing mission, I was not successful with the not awakening Philippe, and when I returned to bed he asked why I had been crying. As I described being tired of being tired and the thoughts that were plaguing me for the past hour, they seemed rather trivial, even to me. I spoke of being so tempted to go on what is now traditional hormone replacement therapy—having made a firm decision to get through this stage of my life using natural methods to help alleviate my chaos—but then remembered that should I get breast cancer, losing sleep wouldn't seem like it was such a horrible option. You see, traditional hormone replacement therapy has been strongly linked to breast cancer, and I have no intention of going there. Besides, said therapy simply delays the chaos of menopause, unless you stay on it forever and ever.

So we talked and then made love—always a good solution to my upsets. But then, of course, I was late getting up and ready for work, so I was in a panic by the time Philippe had to leave, having offered to give me a lift on his way downtown. As was often the case, he had my breakfast in my bowl on the table, my travel mug on the counter, and the yogurt and cream at the ready to allow me to be ready to head to work just as fast as possible. However, when I climbed into his truck I managed to damage my new hose, having worn them for only 3 hours. Once I'd graciously declined his offer to head upstairs to grab a new pair for me, and thus making him late for his own appointment, off we flew, managing a good conversation along the way. It wasn't until I left the truck and neared the Art Gallery that I realized that I'd forgotten to give him a dollar for parking downtown and that I might have left my keys in his truck. I managed to slide in through the outside door behind a co-worker, and then barged my way into another co-worker's office, to sit on a chair and search through my killer large purse for my keys. In the third compartment I checked, there they were! Phew! I wouldn't have to track Philippe down at his hair stylist's salon and ask him to drop off my keys on his way back roughly in my direction. And I wouldn't have to wait for one of my staff members to arrive and let me into my office. So the entire world would not have to know about my most recent bout of menopause-mush-mind! I was saved from further embarrassment, for now!

While I attempt to make light of these situations, particularly for my own well-being, they sure as heck don't feel light when I am in the middle of them. In fact, they make my life seem like a living hell at times, with the sleep deprivation really taking its toll. Perhaps I'm due for yet another trip to my kind and knowledgeable doctor, a woman (most likely of that-certain-age, herself) who specializes in the treatment of menopausal women, of which I most certainly am one. Dr. Pam encourages her patients to research the options that exist to ease the stresses of menopause, and she supports us in our choices, while helping us retain some semblance of sanity. In addition, she provides the medical perspective, and takes care of our bodies, as a whole.

Three cheers for the amazingly supportive people in my life, who put up with my menopause-induced antics!

The Chairs are NOT the Issue

Having settled into my new digs, (a funky, late 1950s or early 1960s apartment, obviously designed by architects on certain substances, based on the lack of 90 degree angles to the walls, the front door located at the side, and the whole building situated askew on the lot), I decided the time had come to give my Muskoka chairs a facelift. They no longer fit in with my color scheme, but I still wanted to use them, cuz, to my way of thinking, the outdoor chairs give the indoor space a neat look.

So I pulled the paint brochures off the bookshelf and re-acquainted myself with the paint colors I'd been pondering for some time, but about which I'd done nothing. Why not try out one of the colors on the chairs, as opposed to jumping right into the major endeavor of painting the entire apartment?

It was "salsa" that leapt out at me. Was this a step back to my former partner, now current friend, from Mexico? Maybe, but the bottom line was that I really liked the color. Besides, I'd already been using and wearing Santa Fe and Mexican colors before I met said Mexican ex, one of the reasons he was attracted to me. Another is that I liked spicy foods. (Note, readers, that these are not good reasons upon which to build a relationship!)

Off I trekked to the local and quaint hardware store to purchase my paint, along with scraping instruments to at least partially remove the traces of previous incarnations from my chairs. They were deck chairs, after all, so why would I bother to properly remove the layers of paint, and the one coat of stain, with chemical remover? I didn't want to have to transport the chairs anywhere to redecorate them. After all, then I'd have to wait for the love o' my life to arrive with his van—a delay that might derail the entire project. And the chemical remover might just kill, or at least cause terrible health side effects for me and my lovely Miss Kitty. Was I justifying not taking the time to do the job right? You bet!

Having purchased my tools, and the paint, in both flat and high gloss versions so I could paint the entire chairs with one and then dapple the finish with another (in the Jacquard style), I wandered home to start my project. Now playing appropriate tunes for the work at hand, I covered the carpet (awful as it was, but it wasn't mine to destroy) and started my scraping and sanding. As always, the time was passing by much more quickly than was the progress of the project at hand. But I was making progress, so I soldiered on.

Then a strange thing happened—particularly strange since I didn't yet know of my menopausal state. I began to cry. No, wait, I should say that I began to sob uncontrollably, to the point where I had to put down my tools, sit down on the floor, and cry. What in the world was going on? I simply was redecorating my Muskoka chairs! I attempted to answer that question, through ramblings and rumblings, which turned into rantings, intermingled with my sobbing. I carried on to the point that my lovely Miss Kitty, awakened from an afternoon nap in the bedroom, made her way down the hall to stand in front of me and stare, somewhat quizzically. So there we sat looking at one another. I then shifted from my ranting and raving approach to the problem, whatever it was, to having a more controlled conversation with the cat, attempting to explain to her what I was feeling and why.

It all boiled down to this: here I was giving these chairs their fourth incarnation, each time in a new partnership, and each time alone. Even the first time, when I had been just recently married, I was decorating my chairs alone. What was my problem? Was I never going to find a partner with whom I would decorate my chairs—you know, together? Was I never again to find myself living with a partner? I was sneaking up on 50 years old and I was decorating my damn chairs alone ... again! Once I'd shouted those statements at Miss Kitty, she up and wandered into the kitchen for a nibble of kibble, my sign that we'd finished our conversation and it was time for me to get back to work.

Menopause or Lunacy

Back to work I got, and soon the whole process of sobbing and carrying on started all over again, and this time I thought my sweet sailor might be home and within range of his telephone ... maybe, just maybe, but doubtful. "I know", I said to myself, "I'll leave a message that I'm thinking of him and I'd love to hear from him when he gets home." So I got control of myself and called this man who I'd been dating for only four months. I became a little less in control when I heard his voicemail greeting, but got things under control. I started to leave my message and managed to sound rather cool, or so I thought, and then something shifted, and I was crying and blathering something about feeling so sad and lonely here working on my chairs. Then, before matters got worse, I gathered myself up and asked him to call me when he could.

To my surprise, he called within an hour, sounding very concerned. He wondered first what had happened. Then, in concerned-guy fashion, he asked if he'd done anything to cause me such an upset. "No!" I assured, and attempted to explain my tears, all the while trying to keep the jerkiness from my voice so he could understand what I was saying. I'm not sure he ever really understood, but he very sweetly offered to abort his boat project and drive in early to see me, instead of waiting until dinner time. I realized instantaneously that I'd like that to happen, but that it would be silly for both of us to get off track with our tasks. But I also realized that because he was concerned (even though he didn't really get it) and because he cared enough to alter his own plans, I now could proceed with my chair decorating and wait to see this pretty darn cool man later that evening, when we'd have dinner, some wine, and probably some good lovin'. That's all I had needed. So I explained that I'd be okay and that we both needed to get back to work, and thanked him so much for caring. My very puzzled Philippe then hung up and we both returned to our projects.

I must confess that a few tears fell on and off throughout the rest of the afternoon, until I readied myself for my sweetie-pie's arrival. But mostly I considered my strong reaction to redecorating these bloody chairs alone, once again, and what they represented. Most importantly, I'd made it through another of my strange, huge mood swings. I'd felt comfortable seeking Philippe's help in getting to the other side of this moment of despair and he'd responded lovingly. So all would be well and I'd face my painting task the next day with much more strength—and ideally, with much more level-headedness.

Watch Out for Your Job...
and for Your Self-Esteem

Prior to realizing I was edging toward menopause, and having just relocated from my home turf in southern Ontario, I accepted a position with a small organization that seemed to fit very well with my background. This position was new within the charity, and was a new focus for me, so I found myself on less than solid ground. In addition, having worked in a feminist-based organization for close to a decade, I found working within a male (in fact, patriarchal- beyond- belief) system a considerable challenge. But before even beginning the job, I had contributed to an application that had resulted in a considerable grant for the organization, so I felt I had made a good start. Had I only known!

As I settled into my work, I made excellent connections within the fundraising community and with our supporters, and secured some healthy revenues. But I sensed something unhealthy going on around me, which culminated in the abrupt departure of our executive director, my female boss, with whom I thought I'd established a good and enjoyable relationship. Then, when I was asked to step in and keep the ship afloat until the Board of Directors considered their next steps, I became excited by the challenge, knowing that I was capable and well qualified to take the helm of this organization and move it forward, with an emphasis on public education. But my excitement wore thin as the months (and then years) rolled by with me attempting to cover two jobs, and finding myself in a position of holding a large amount of responsibility, but with no authority. When I tried to make changes that would get the charity better known, my wings were clipped, and I was reminded of my place within the organization (although it was anything but defined). And any time I took suggestions to the Board for their consideration, they were put on the back burner, unless they entailed me taking on more work to make something exciting happen, for which the Board members generally took the credit. But determined to do good work in the community, I toughed it out, kept my chin up, swallowed my pride, pandered to the male Board members, and got the job done. Thank goodness for the two female Board members who supported me and my ideas, or I'd have gone stark raving mad even sooner than I did.

Without dragging you through all the details, suffice it to say that, as I attempted to work through this situation and prove myself worthy of the position of Executive Director, I was alternatively encouraged and then put in my place, to the point that I hesitated to move forward on any of my ideas. And so I learned to work very closely with the female Board members, and to couch my ideas as theirs, so they would be thought worthy of consideration. The result, on a long-term basis, was the total devastation of my self-esteem and self-confidence, to the point that I became paralyzed, with the Board then having some proof that I was unable to direct the organization. And after a long and extremely agonizing process, I experienced what amounted to a constructive dismissal, and found myself out of work.

On the positive side, however, something snapped within me during this process, in the midst of my menopausal mush-mindedness, and I mustered up the strength to "stand up and fight and be counted". It was an applicable paraphrase that I clearly remember from a song back in the day. But of course I can't remember the title or who recorded it. So much for the English major being able to cite her source!

And further, on the bright side, during those few years I connected with several people in the community who were thrilled when I developed the will to fight to take care of myself, and who recommended the appropriate professional services, resulting in this sordid tale having a partially happy ending for me. In fact, through it all I formed a friendship with the incoming executive director, who is a really good person, and who I now consider a very good friend.

Looking back at it all, I have no doubt that I would have handled this situation very differently had I not been brand-new to the community and ramping up to menopause, and therefore full of self doubt and the chaos of constantly having to recover from the effects of my impaired memory. I'm convinced that many women at this stage of life who encounter this type of abusive treatment at work, and who are not lucky enough to have developed such solid sources of help, fall by the wayside in numbers large enough to be alarming, if we knew the statistics. You see, this is the type of experience that can stomp you down to the point that you can't take care of yourself, and so you accept your fate and continue your life in a diminished capacity...and you never tell anyone your tale because you feel you brought it on yourself and so deserved it. When I look at the times in women's lives when they reach the so called "glass ceiling" and settle for lower-level career positions than they'd been striving for, and in some cases had achieved, I can't help but notice it happens in their mid-forties, just about the time when many women are heading into menopause, but don't yet know it. Coincidence? I think not!

Menopause Killed the Cat—Almost

My eyes opened and there it was—the horror of dealing with the cat. If it weren't for dear, sweet Stinky Monkey, I'd have been freed of cat-care once Miss Kitty moved on to kitty heaven. But no! I had to get a "little sister" for the old doll, and thus extended this hell called "kitty motherhood", complete with the damn responsibility of finding a sitter for her whenever I wanted to spend time away from home. Now boating season was upon us, finally, after a long period of crappy weather, and here I was worrying about finding a kitty sitter, when I should have been getting some work done before packing to head out for an extra-long weekend.

Yes, I knew that I'd been taking her to Philippe's with me and things had been working out quite nicely, even though she was still a little freaked by the whole travel and new digs thing. But why the hell was she such a "fraidy-cat"? She was nervous and she made me nervous. Even though Philippe said he'd become quite comfortable having her at his place, I suspected he really hated her being there. Oh, the trauma of trying to figure out what to do! I was sure, also that she'd not settled into being an only kitty, and that she looked for Miss Kitty all the time, still—even under the stove and behind the fridge, although I'm sure she'd never, ever seen Miss Kitty in those places. Oh, the poor wee thing. No doubt she'd be better off somewhere else—with a kitty mom that didn't abandon her or drag her somewhere all the time.

Yeah, that was it! She'd be perfect with an older woman who sits a lot and would love to have a kitty curled up on her lap and keeping her company and warm. Oh, wouldn't that be the ideal life for Stinky? "Hey, maybe Philippe's mom", I thought. "She's in the garden a lot, but when she comes in at night, wouldn't she love to have Stinky greet her and spend the evening in her lap?" Oh yes, I was sure she would. But wait a minute. We'd talked about that when I thought Miss Kitty needed a new home, before deciding on adopting Stinky Monkey, and she wasn't at all convinced that she wanted to enter into kitty motherhood again. "Okay, so there's my mom, now that she's close by rather than almost across the country", I reasoned. "She still misses her critters terribly, and I know she'd love to have Stinky with her." I thought so. I could check. "Now, she does have Cullen down there an awful lot, and Stinky doesn't like kids", I remembered. "But she doesn't hurt them—in fact, she hides from them, so that shouldn't pose a problem." Then there were all those knick-knacks on her windowsills. They'd have to be cleared away, at least from one window. But the last time we had talked, Mom thought she liked life without worrying about pets, especially with grandson Cullen so close by, and her walking him twice a day and entertaining him often in her own digs. And that wee guy sure did need entertaining. "Rats, I'll bet she doesn't want any part of it", I concluded, as all these thoughts whirled around my confused and distraught brain.

I let myself fall back into the couch. What was I to do with this overwhelming situation? I wanted it solved once and for all, and I wanted it solved before we left for our weekend, the next morning.

Suddenly, I had a moment of clarity. Yes, that was it! How could I have missed the obvious for this long? "I'll simply have her put to sleep", I reasoned. That would do it. I'd never have to worry if she was doing okay with someone else, or if she was being treated right. No, there was nothing wrong with her health, and she was really not a difficult cat to deal with; but damn it, she'd been so anxious and unhappy since Miss Kitty died. Yes indeed, she, too, would be far better off in kitty heaven. We could bury her beside her big sister and they would be happy together, and not causing anyone any trouble.

With that problem solved, I called the vet's office and talked with Catherine, the veterinary assistant. She was shocked, having just seen me go through the hell of making the decision around Miss Kitty, and then hearing me make such a fast (possibly rash?) decision about Stinky. But as she said, I knew her best, and if she'd been displaying signs of such nervousness and discomfort, then so be it. But no, the doctor had no time until the next afternoon. Drat! That was no good. I had to deal with this situation today. So I told her I'd call back. No problem! I then struggled to remember the name of the emergency vet clinic where Miss Kitty was put to sleep, to make an appointment with them. Well, what a shock it was when the woman there informed me that I'd have to make an appointment with the vet to discuss the situation, before bringing in a completely healthy animal for euthanasia. How dare they? After all, this was my cat and my decision. But not to be thwarted, I called my house-call, homeopathic vet and left her a message. She'd understand the sound reasoning behind my decision.

By the time the phone rang and it was the house-call vet calling back, I was immersed, finally, in working to get things accomplished for my clients before I left for the extended weekend. And Philippe had called and I'd told him that I was thinking about finding Stinky a home. No I didn't tell him I was thinking about killing her—that truth was too difficult for me to admit. Philippe's reaction was one of shock and disbelief, given I truly loved Stinky and enjoyed having her in my life. "But I know you really don't like having her at your place", I asserted, with him replying and setting the record straight.

"I have absolutely no problem having her here!"

"But, you don't want her on the boat ever again, even though she didn't cause any trouble", I blurted in response.

"That's not it", Philippe explained, "I just think she's not at all comfortable and that you don't relax either, when she's with us."

"But what about if she were to pull the carpet with her claws, like she did your area rug at home? You were so angry about that," I asked, already having anticipated the trouble without it having occurred.

"Well, I hadn't thought of that." Then silence. So there it was—he didn't want her on board. "But I don't think she'll do that, especially if you bring something for her to scratch, like she has at home."

Oh of course, it was back to me taking all the responsibility again, I thought to myself, and before I could take that thought further, Philippe suggested we give her a try that weekend and see how she did, given the seas looked like they should be calm.

So when Dr. Lesley called, I already was quite relaxed, and she calmed me with her quiet respect for the kitty-mother and kitty relationship. She asked what Stinky was up to that made me feel she was really unhappy and stressed, and then explained that it would take her a long time to adjust to life without Miss Kitty, given that was pretty much all she'd known. I described her nervous behavior and her fear when I was getting ready to go away, knowing that I'd soon grab her and shove her into her carrying case. The good doctor recommended that I use some of the homeopathic remedies I most likely still had around the house to help Miss Kitty feel calm during her final weeks of life, and she recommended a cat pheromone spray that helps cats adjust to new situations. This made sense to me. So I was back to my other vet's office to ask if they carry the spray, explaining that I was now down off the ceiling and looking for solutions other than killing the cat. No, they didn't have any, but Catherine recommended a couple of vet clinics for me to call. Then the emergency vet clinic called and I explained what I had in mind, and the woman there seemed very relieved. She assured me the spray would help. So I called the one location in town that she thought might have it in stock and, sure enough, they did. I arranged to have some set aside for me to pick up on my way out of town, and proceeded to settle in and finish my work, and then to pack up me and Stinky and leave for Philippe's digs, before heading out on the boat the next morning.

Stinky did join us on the trip. And even when, about 50 minutes out from the yacht club, I found myself in the terrible position of announcing to Philippe that we had to head back because I'd forgotten the kitty litter and box, I felt happy that Stinky was with us. While Philippe wasn't thrilled about turning back and losing the favorable tide, turn back he did. Once he returned from his digs with the forgotten essential items, we had a nice lunch and I served him a beer. Before long, all was well and I thanked him for his efforts to have Stinky aboard. She had a pretty good weekend, and the pheromone spray was quite effective.

Part way through the trip when she was sleeping beside me, and then again when we'd arrived home and she was sleeping on my lap, I marveled that the trauma and panic created by my menopausal state almost prompted me to kill my cat. In this case, it would not have been curiosity that killed the cat, but that damn stage of life called menopause that was the culprit!

You know, thinking back, I'll bet my vet's office did have space that day, but Catherine was protecting me, and Stinky Monkey, from the ravages of insanity—mine, not the cat's. Hey, maybe Catherine has a mother, an aunt, a sister, or a friend who is going crazy with menopause, and she knew that if she could get me through this particular crisis, Stinky Monkey would live to settle into the boating life, and I'd recover to tell the story of when menopause almost killed the cat.

Fighting the "Has-Been" Feeling

The feeling strikes me when I read my alumni magazines. The feeling strikes me when I watch special programs on television about the past, present, and future of the National Ballet of Canada and the dedication of young people to stay focused on their passions. The feeling strikes me whenever I come face-to-face with a young person, in particular, who is thriving in a field in which she or he had dreamed of succeeding...when I come face to face with *any* people who are living their dreams... or even when I encounter a young person who seems amazingly together at a very early age.

I feel like a "has-been", or perhaps more accurately, a "never-was". But, I'm not really a "never-was", because I lived an amazing decade when I was fighting the good fight for Planned Parenthood Waterloo Region and completely revamping the 1-800- infosex line for Planned Parenthood Ontario. During that time, I gained a mind-boggling amount of experience, set in an exciting background of living life as an advocate for women's right to choose, a teacher of healthy sexuality, an executive director of two small charities, and a fundraiser for an exceptional cause. In the midst of it all, I had the pleasure of interacting with media outlets throughout Ontario, and lobbying provincial and federal politicians to save sexual health funding from the chopping block. Come to think of it, perhaps I am a "peaked-too-early" person, so have spent the rest of my time looking for a follow-up to that amazing early life experience.

I'm a person who has lived a life of going with the flow. I'm a person who has not formulated many dreams to follow. But I am a person who is adaptable and who does reasonably well at whatever I decide to do at any given time, often with little or no formal education in the area of my pursuits. I seem to be a jack of all trades and a master of none. Therefore, often I feel like a fake—like someone who always pretends to know what she's doing and often lives in fear of being found out. But the longer I live, the more I realize that many of us live our lives in that way, with some faking it better than others. Coming into menopause—a time of passage in a woman's life—has heightened my feelings of faking it, while leaving me with much less energy to play a convincing role. This lack of energy, coupled with my sketchy memory, leads me into panic situations, when I simply can't draw from my memory bank enough information to allow me to keep up the pretence. Many times, I simply want to run away from any situation in which I find myself caught between a rock and a hard place. Then I realize that I have lived enough life and gained enough experience to pull it off, to truly know what I am speaking about, and that I am experienced enough to have come extremely close to achieving expertise in many areas, albeit by osmosis.

In my less frazzled moments, I see that the trick to finding my next riveting cause or path will be to follow my heart, use my brains to know it when it comes my way, and capitalize on the opportunities it provides. Yes that's definitely the ticket!

It Can't be Getting Worse, Can it?

Just when you think you're in the clear, suddenly it seems you're getting worse. Or maybe not really getting worse, but that you've been thrown right back into the thick of it. It's like some sick power from somewhere is toying with you and having fun reminding you just how bad it can be. Mind you, the upside of these reminders is that, once they pass, you do get the chance to realize that you truly have "come a long way, baby". Okay, enough with the cryptic stuff. Let me explain.

My sweetie-pie had been sick for almost a week, and about two days into his nasty cold, I started feeling crappy. So simultaneously, I was doing the nursemaid thing, given he was in much worse shape than was I. Then, just as I was thinking I was out of the woods, and when he was definitely on the mend, I awakened feeling like I was in relapse mode. I was cranky, disappointed, and frustrated, and I hadn't yet made my morning latte when the phone rang. I noticed on call display that it was my chiropractor calling, and thought that maybe he was checking to see if the sailor man and I were feeling well enough to make our dinner date with him and his wife, two days hence. So as cheerfully as possible, I answered the phone. It was the morning receptionist asking how I was doing, and then pausing as if for me to continue the conversation. When I didn't take the bait, she nicely advised me that she thought they had me booked for an appointment for such-and-such a time that morning, and did they have it wrong? "Oh damn", says I, "you probably have it right, and I've probably forgotten ... I'm so sorry." Of course, she accepted my apology and asked if I wanted to rebook, which I did for later that same day. Again, I apologized profusely, feeling like an idiot and feeling badly because of the lack of respect I was showing them for wasting their time.

Wandering back to the kitchen to create my latte, I commented to Philippe that the call was from Jeff's office and that I had missed an appointment with him for 8:45 that morning, and that I felt terrible about standing him up. I do believe I also mumbled something about not believing that I didn't clue in when I saw on the display that the call was from his office. Then, all of a sudden, I was standing in the kitchen crying. I don't mean I had a few tears in my eyes. I mean I was crying, like I'd just been informed of the death of my best and last friend. And there's my sweet man, looking at me with such concern in his eyes, asking what's happened, had he done or said something to upset me, had I hurt myself somehow, etc. Then, when I looked up, pathetically no doubt, and said, "I don't know what's wrong", he reached out and held me tight.

"Oh", he said, and that was all he needed to say. Because right then we both realized I was having another one of those moments. Yes, I was having a relapse, and I am sure he was thinking what I was thinking: thank goodness, this kind of behavior had become the exception instead of the norm!

So with more hugs and a smooch or two...and one of his rare and cherished "I love you" offerings, off he went to his shop, and there I was, left to make my latte and to wonder what the hell had happened, and to finish my release of frustrations through crying. How the heck did I get from learning that I'd missed my chiropractic appointment to feeling like my world was ending?

With my latte made, off I toddled to my desk and computer, and set about my workday. But I just wasn't settled enough emotionally yet to focus on my tasks at hand. So I responded to some email messages. One was from a former colleague and treasured friend, updating me on the latest in the saga of our former place of employment, a wonderful little charitable organization which we'd helped build to a place of strength before moving on to other things. Recently, it had come to light that it was in financial trouble, and the current administration was considering actions with which we did not agree, so we were trying to help resolve the situation. As I read her message, it dawned on me that the situation was a huge source of stress for me, and that I was feeling like a child of mine was dying. So I sat back, sipped on my latte, and allowed myself to acknowledge how this stress was impacting me. Then, on I plodded with email messages and there was one from another very good friend from that era and that organization. Reading her message, I decided to tell her, in complete confidence, about the situation with our pet charity, and as I wrote, my message grew in length and all my current stresses poured out of me. When I was finished confessing my sins—er, my stresses, I mean—I sipped the last of my latte and was ready to start my workday.

So yes, sometimes it does seem as though it can be getting worse, or at least like you've had a huge relapse. But at least for me, these moments are now much easier to handle than were the earlier traumas, or, perhaps I should say that the complete distress lasts only a relatively short time. And I'm able to handle them with clarity and from a position of strength. Hey, perhaps the saying is right, that what doesn't kill you makes you strong. For a long while, through my menopausal carryings-on, I was sure that my brother's version of that adage was the correct one: what doesn't kill you drags you through such hell that you are left exhausted and irreparably damaged. Forgive me dear bro, if I've completely bastardized your oh-so brilliant adage, but I think I've captured the sentiment.

Jottings

A Mind Blowing Experience

The mental changes and challenges
during the menopausal years

Confessions of a Formerly Organized Woman

"You're right," said a good friend a few years my senior. "Those of us who are perennially disorganized can roll with the punches, whereas those of you who once were organized must feel extremely frustrated and confused." Once again, I thank the goddesses for women friends who understand my plight as I struggle through yet another exasperating experience in a day in the life of a menopausal moron.

No, wait a minute. Author and amazing woman Louise Hay tells me I'm not supposed to put myself down like this. However, how can one always be a good girl and follow Ms. Hay's wise advice when she feels like her mind has vacated her body? Given the things she does, and perhaps more devastating, the things she doesn't know she's done, she finds herself in a state of panic and has to dig deep and painfully pour over the chain of events that might, just might, help her pull together the pieces of the puzzle.

Okay, let me explain a little more clearly what I mean by all this cryptic blathering.

The day was going along swimmingly well. I was working like a mad woman and getting duties ticked off my list of things to do. I love it when that happens—I feel so damn accomplished. Yes, it is the A-type person I am. And that's where I think I run into trouble. Because I am an A-type person, I have extremely high expectations of myself and am totally and completely thrown into a panic when I fall short. Wait a minute; I've become cryptic again, haven't I? Sorry about that—I'll get back to my story now.

The day was going along swimmingly well. I was working like a mad woman and getting duties ticked off my list of things to do. Next on the list was for me to pull together a package for a potential client, complete with copies of some profiles I'd written many years ago. Having very recently made some copies of these articles for other packages, I reached into the file drawer, expecting the originals of these profiles to be at my fingertips at the front of the appropriate file. Well, you can imagine the shock and horror I felt when I didn't find the profiles where they ought to be! If you are an A-type perfectionist who likes things *just so*, you'll be able to imagine my emotional response. "Where have I put them?" I asked myself. "I so clearly remember placing them back in this file, where they belong, because they are my only originals and so very important to me". Not only was I missing the profiles themselves, but also the thank you letters from those people I profiled—a very valuable combination. Indeed, I could feel my heart start to beat faster, and my breaths become shallow and rapid. I had to slow myself down, think, and look. Yes, I had to keep looking, because I so clearly remembered returning these documents to this file.

After several minutes of dedicated and somewhat panicked searching, I finally resigned myself to the fact that I had not returned the documents to the appropriate file. So where did I last have them? Where could I have left them? How could I leave them somewhere when they were so important to me? "Stop, wait a minute", I insisted quietly to myself. "You're falling back into the pattern of denigrating yourself—a behavior that helps nothing and serves only to make you feel crappy." So I took several deep breaths, remembered what Louise Hay had to say about pulling one's self out of these situations, and began retracing the steps of that day when I had made the most recent set of copies. Yes, that was it! I had made those copies at the office of a client, who generously allowed me to use her organization's photocopier. Surely, I didn't leave them there. I couldn't have, could I? Surely not! Oh no, I didn't mail them along with the photocopies, did I? Oh no, oh no, oh no! Now chill out, Donna Faye, and think hard. Perhaps they were at Philippe's place, because I stayed there that weekend. Now stay out of that downward spiral and figure out this mystery.

Well, emailing my client can't hurt, particularly since she also is a friend. Yes, that's where I'll start. So email the client I did, explaining my dilemma, and asking her if she'd seen them, and if not I'd check at Philippe's. And because she's a friend I indicated my frustration with having once been an amazingly organized person and now, thanks to menopause-mush- mind, I found myself in these horrible situations in which I was trying desperately to figure out what I'd done with something I desperately did not want to lose, all the while raking myself over the coals. She assured me that they were on her desk and that she had enjoyed reading them. She also assured me I was not insane and offered me that bit of wisdom found at the beginning of this little tale of woe.

While I felt much relieved knowing the whereabouts of my important documents, I felt extremely frustrated that I'd wasted a good 45 minutes of my previously productive day. And as the day progressed, I felt even more frustrated that this upsetting event adversely affected the balance of a day that had started so darn well. You see, I never really got back on track after experiencing yet another incidence of menopause mush mind.

Oh the horror—the horror of it all!

Am I Budgeting-Inept or Is This Menopause?

A sad tale of me, money, and menopause-mush-mind

Off the top, let me be clear that working within a balanced budget ceased to be my forte some time ago, and became increasingly worse as easy-to-acquire credit and debit cards came along. And because I'd always managed to make regular payments, my credit rating made me attractive to lenders. After all, I've been an excellent, reliable source of interest income for them, so why wouldn't they want to lend me more money?

At this particular juncture in my life, when my credit card balance had grown uncomfortably high, and I'd paid off a chunk of my past sins loan, I was tired of being "highly leveraged" and finally wanted to get my financial act together. So we (my financial planner and I) decided to consolidate my debt into a lower-interest loan, and lower my credit card limit. Good plan, I felt, and an effective way for me to improve my financial health. (You see, when you spend much of your adult life working for good, but poor-paying, causes in the not-for-profit sector, your own profit margin tends to take a bit of a beating—especially when you are the only bread winner in your family. At least, that's my story and I'm sticking to it!)

So the consolidation loan came through and the money was sitting in my bank account. I excitedly sat down in front of my computer to transfer enough money into my credit card account to pay off that baby. I wished with all my heart that I could be doing it with my own money, rather than with more money from the bank, albeit at a much lower interest rate than said bank was charging me on my card. Self-ridicule aside, I guided myself through the steps necessary to make this transfer of money on my online banking system, and shut down my computer feeling rather smug. I would check in a couple of days, and would see a zero balance on my credit card, and I would curb my spending habits and watch the balance of my "big loan" decrease. And I would feel much better about my self-discipline.

As promised, two days later, I checked my credit card balance to see absolutely no change, even though the payment amount had been removed from my checking account. Shocked and disappointed, I shut down the system and determined I would check again the next day. The next day came and I was greeted with the same reality. I became quite concerned, but decided to give it one more day before panicking. On the third day, when no change in my credit card balance had occurred, panic I did. I called the credit card people and explained the situation, and was told I would receive a call back. So I waited...and waited...and waited. When the call came, I learned that I had paid the money to the telephone company, in error. I couldn't imagine how I could have been so careless and stupid, and that the telephone company could have accepted that amount of money without question. Did they think I was planning on making an enormous change in my calling patterns, like calling Russia on a daily basis, or some such thing?

Upon inquiring what to do next, I was given another number to call, a local one. Apparently, this person would instruct me on how I could set about retrieving my money from the phone people and getting it off to my credit card account, where it belonged. The woman who greeted me on the phone was extremely pleasant and helpful, and before long, we had the steps in place to correct my embarrassing error. Before ending our conversation, I thanked the wonderful woman profusely, and explained that this was just one more mistake induced by my current condition called menopause-mush-mind. Well, she chuckled heartily and spoke of her all-too-clear understanding of my current state of mind. We conversed on the topic of menopause for several minutes, during which time I told her that my plan was to write a book with a humorous slant about the *joys* of menopause, and that this episode of banking-ineptitude most certainly would find its way into the collection of the assorted tales of my menopause experience. I'm sure you will appreciate my delight when this faceless confidante exclaimed with great pleasure that I must do just that, because thousands of women will benefit from my humorous approach to this sometimes very deflating and depressing topic.

So here I am doing just that, and sometimes still struggling with my financial situation, but making progress. Looking back, I realize that spending had become therapeutic for me (yes, the old retail therapy situation). Every item of clothing, footwear, and jewelry that I purchased seemed worth the debt because it made me feel good about myself for at least a short time. And although I don't recommend that route, I now see a benefit in it, in that I have accumulated so much *stuff* that I don't feel the need to shop and buy, because I keep uncovering and enjoying items I'd forgotten I'd purchased, so feel like I have brand new things.

Perhaps this is a new twist on reduce, reuse, recycle!

Menopause—The Perfect Time to Work on Your Own...From Home

Yes, I have to admit that it sounded a tad crazy. But what was I to do? My maternity leave contract had ended and the best-laid plans for me to stay on in a part-time capacity had gone sideways. Most certainly, the thought of going out and looking for employment seemed at once daunting and nauseating. So here was the opportunity for which I'd been waiting and couldn't pass up—here was a contract lucrative enough to get me started in my own business. And I seemed to have the faith to believe that I'd be able to swing it.

But what about the fact that I couldn't seem to keep track of my own finances, much less the financial arrangements for a consulting business? What about the fact that I seemed to need a push to work each day, provided, or so I thought, only by heading into an office and having to answer to a boss? Okay, well, the first "what about" could be a problem; however, the second "what about" could be solved by thinking of my clients as my bosses. And the thought of being my own boss and working from home seemed so compelling that I simply had to make it happen. So there I was, creating my company name, my business cards, my letterhead, and my sales pitch. And there I was, landing my first year-long contract and working on another contract that could lead to a long-term one. The next thing I knew, I saw my ad in the newspaper and, low and behold, I was running my own business!

So the plan was to keep my nose to the grind stone and, given I no longer needed to dress up for work each day, I could stop buying clothing and jewelry and thus keep myself in a pretty good financial position, remembering that nothing was certain in this world of consulting. Well, the first month went pretty well and then I decided I needed different home office furniture, given that the small writing desk I had been using just wasn't cutting it. Then, there was the computer situation that had raised its ugly head, and the need for a new computer arose. Oh yes, then the new office chair turned out to be detrimental to my physical well being, so why not buy the one I'd always wanted, particularly given its ergonomic benefits. Oh and my new hobby of belly dancing needed new clothing to go with it, especially if I was to perform, which I really wanted to do. And while I didn't need very many new clothes, the old ones really were old and, in many cases, didn't fit so well anymore. So the only way to cull what no longer worked was to buy some wonderful consignment shop clothing, which, inevitably, needed some new jewels to make them happen for me.

The second contract materialized because I did a damn fine job with the short-term contract. And so it kept going. And then one day, I understood the very reason why I needed to make this consulting business work. Okay, so there was one reason that was really important for me, and that was that it allowed me the freedom to become a published writer. And there was a second and equally important reason—one that applied to many women of my age and stage.

We all know that a major downside of menopause is the accompanying hot flashes that render one incapable of avoiding pulling off layers of clothing in the middle of the day, no matter where we are located at the time. So by working at home, we menopausal maniacs could merrily disrobe while working away in our home offices, and no one would be the wiser, except maybe our pets. Yes indeed, working from home seems to be the key to enduring those all-consuming and most uncomfortable eruptions within us that result in every cell in our body perspiring and the feeling that we will spontaneously combust. Oh what a relief to be in my home office and feel free to fling off the majority, or all, of my clothing and then continue to work! So when discussing business on the telephone with a menopausal woman, do try to avoid thinking that she may be stark naked. Whether or not this thought intrigues you, just don't go there. It almost certainly will take your mind off the business at hand, and will lead you to places you really shouldn't go, if you are to continue to deal with this woman in a professional manner.

Rex Forgotten

Many Canadians reading this story will know about Rex Murphy, that rather unusual looking, very bright, and extremely articulate Canadian Broadcasting Corporation host with the prominent eyes; but, more importantly, the very bright man with the most interesting insights. And here was Rex coming to "the island"—yes, Vancouver Island, and I had an opportunity to buy tickets to see him. Yes indeed, I told my friend who worked for the college sponsoring the event, I'd buy at least one ticket from her, but I wanted to check with a friend or two first to see if they'd want to join me. Oh this would be the perfect way to get back into the intellectual scene and to plunge into thinking about national, and maybe even global matters, instead of simply dwelling on my own issues.

Diligently I set about asking a few people I thought might want to join me to hear Rex and to engage in some rousing discussion thereafter. But alas, everyone was busy or simply not as interested in Rex as was I. So no problem, I'd go on my own, assured to know at least one person there—my friend from whom I was buying the ticket. Excellent! This would be fun.

Many weeks later, there was a message from this friend, which I opened with great excitement. As I waited for the message to appear on my laptop screen, I suddenly started thinking about not having heard back from her about my Rex ticket, and then not remembering ever talking with her about tickets. How long ago did all that happen? When was the date of Rex's talk? Well, by the time I finished searching my poor brain for all those questions and answers, there was the message on the computer screen, encouraging me to attend the next in their series of lectures—yes, that same series in which Rex was speaking, or, it seemed, had already spoken.

So I quickly moved to reply to my friend's message, typing only, "Oh no, have I missed Rex?"

With disappointment pending, I sent my message, and within minutes, I received my answer. "Yes, and he was excellent. But not to worry, come to this next one—she'll be amazing."

Oh no! I'd done it again. In the muddle of my menopause-mush-mind, I'd forgotten about something quite important to me, and I hadn't even realized I'd forgotten about it until I received something to jolt my ailing brain cells into gear. But I didn't rant or rave or create a scene. With resignation on a happening now far too familiar, I typed a meek apology for not following up on buying my ticket, and then asked my friend to

Menopause or Lunacy

save one for me for the upcoming lecture. I assured her that this time I'd written the event into my daybook along with a note to take money to pay for it at our next meeting. This time I would remember, provided I remembered to look at my daybook.

I almost liked it better when I still had been upset enough by my brain-deadness to kick up a fuss and rant and rave and carry on. This resignation was most disconcerting. Was it true then that one doesn't really recover from menopause, but instead becomes used to its symptoms and resigns oneself to learning to live with the situation or, perhaps more accurately, used to living with the disappointment?

But then, a bit of panic set in. If I could so thoroughly forget about going to hear politically astute Rex Murphy, could I not just as easily forget about something very important in my work life now that I was working on my own as a consultant, without a solid infrastructure to help me keep on top of things? I mean, I realize that I sometimes forget to check my daybook. And I feel extremely relieved when I do check it and no disaster has taken place, like me forgetting an appointment or a report deadline. So what would happen if, when I did remember to check my schedule, I had forgotten something very important and it led to a client no longer wanting my services?

"Now settle down, Donna", I told myself. My saving grace seemed to be my somewhat photographic memory.

Once I'd written down an important appointment in my daybook, I could visualize the page and at least remember that something was written in a certain spot (on which day of the week, and in the morning, afternoon, or evening). I would check the book and figure out where I needed to be or what I needed to do. I felt momentary relief, until I realized that I'd forgotten Rex because I'd forgotten to write him into my book, so when I looked at the two-page per week spread there was nothing there to see, so there was nothing there to remember. Ugh!

Yes, indeed, poor Rex hadn't made it into the book, so he had become Rex forgotten. I'm sure he'd suffered worst fates than this one, but I sure was disappointed. Surely, the point was that I needed to figure out a way to remind myself to not forget to write down appointments. Maybe technology was the answer to my memory loss and working around it. Perhaps I needed to purchase the perfect electronic planner and all would be well, except, of course, if I forgot to turn it on and refer to it. Perhaps I could make a note—but where could I place the note where I would remember to look at it, in order to remember to look at my new and fancy day planner?

Oh, it is all too frazzling just thinking about it, and I must stop. So far, as long as I'd remembered to buy the tickets and write the thing into the good book, all was well. So far. And suddenly, just as I was about to give up on the whole idea, I had it: I would write a note to myself on a sticky note and stick it to my bathroom mirror, to remember to check my daybook each morning through the week, and to check it on Friday afternoon for the next week, so as to not miss anything on the Monday. Yes, that was it! Now if I can only remember to write the sticky note!

In the meantime, Rex, please accept my apologies for not keeping our date, which had never really become a date that I had to remember.

In Search of a Brain—Ideally Mine

Once upon a time, I had a brain and a memory—that worked. Alas, it seems that both assets of mine have diminished almost to the point of total depletion. To illustrate this rather dramatic assertion, I invite you to join me in taking a look at a single example in a morning of my new life, and let's keep in mind that since I entered my menopausal journey, any day of my life can contain many such frustrating and aggravating experiences.

While luxuriating in the cockpit of *Euphoria*, Philippe's and my sailboat, in the beautiful area of British Columbia known as Desolation Sound, I remembered (now this, in itself, was a feat of remarkable proportions) that I'd finished the film in my camera the day before. So I found my camera (yet another amazing feat for so early in the morning) and removed the exposed film. To my amazement, I easily located a new film, loaded it into the camera, placed the exposed film in the canister from the new film, and then attempted to place this exposed film with the other exposed film I'd stored several days previously. Now I'm sure you'll grant me that this task should be a relatively simple one. Those of us with brains that work would have placed the previously exposed film in a logical and safe place. And those of us with memories that work would have remembered, without difficulty, the location of that place. One of my wonderful female friends, closer to the other side of her menopausal journey, has begun to refer to her memory as her "forgettery". I do believe she's found the perfect way to describe how totally and completely our memories can fail us during this stage of our lives…and perhaps beyond! So back to the current story. To my backpack I went, to what I thought was a very logical and safe place for my exposed films, planning to place the one item with its sister item. However, I could not find the first exposed film. Now the problem with this very good backpack was that it contained way too many pockets for a menopausal woman who can't hope to remember their locations. Patiently (at first), I searched through every pocket in the backpack, starting at the front and going on through to the back—and back again to the front. By this time, my patience was wearing thin and I could feel the tears welling up in my eyes. I simply hate feeling stupid, something I seem to do on a regular basis these days.

It was as I started rifling through the garbage that my sweet Philippe realized I was having another menopausal moment, and chose, wisely, to stay out of my way. When he could no longer stand the fussing and the sighing (yes, very heavy sighing), he suggested that I'd obviously chosen a very safe place for the film in question. Perhaps, just perhaps, if I called off the intense search, which was getting me nowhere at the moment, the stash of films would surface at another time, mostly likely before our trip was over. About to protest, I shut my mouth, choked back some tears, heeded his good advice, and we got on with the day.

Why the tears over something so silly, you might ask. Well, for me it is that feeling of having absolutely no recollection of the events leading up to losing something important to me that drives me right 'round the bend and off the deep end. In the past, when both my brain and memory were my constant companions, I could work back through my memory and trace my actions that led to placing a certain item in a certain place. In fact, I often coached others on this systematic process to help them recover that which was lost! While I still seem to be able to guide others (because their own brains are still working), I cannot, for the life of me, do the same for myself. These days, no matter how long I sit and try to envision when I last held an item in question—an act that used to lead me to quickly find it—almost always, my mind remains blank. (Worse still, I'll remember something very clearly but, as it turns out, erroneously, as I discover when I find the item in a place completely different than where I clearly remembered placing it.) As these experiences of incorrect recollection have become more prevalent, quite often I can reason with myself that this type of behavior does not mean I've become a complete idiot. But sometimes I still become totally frustrated and incensed that I, a formerly intelligent and sharp-brained person, now forget even the simplest and most basic bits and pieces of information that help sane people keep their lives in order.

Fear not! Those who have gone before me through this rite of passage tell me that life returns to relative normalcy and, in fact, we end up stronger for having survived our menopausal years! I can't say I believe them just yet, but perhaps I will one day forget how bad things used to be. Now that particular act of forgetting most certainly will be a blessing, rather than a curse!

A Change in Perspective about a Dear Old Friend

I never cease to be amazed at how moving through menopause, a major rite of passage in a woman's life, can offer a change in perspective in any number of life's issues. Such an issue in my life was the advancing age of my "old doll"—my aged Siamese princess kitty, who suffered a major health set back.

During what I thought would be a routine yearly visit to the vet to have my two cats, Miss Kitty and Skinky Monkey, receive a physical examination and their annual shots, I mentioned that Miss Kitty, the old doll, seemed to be chewing on any manner of paper. That's when the blur started. The next thing I knew, I was agreeing to a major collection of blood tests. By way of the test results, the vet would determine if Miss K was strong enough for the dental surgery she needed, in order to alleviate the discomfort and pain in her mouth and to stop the bacteria produced by the tooth decay and plaque build-up that contributed to her kidney weakness.

"How the hell did all this happen?" I found myself asking the vet, and still am not at all sure of the answer

I received. However, I am sure about the extent to which the Miss Kitty saga lightened my wallet considerably.

From that time forward until Miss Kitty's death, her dive into poor kitty health was steep. There was the blood work; then the dental surgery; the change of diet resulting in me begging and pleading with the old doll to eat, in order to ingest her antibiotics; the two near-death experiences caused by extreme dehydration; the administration of fluids underneath the sweet kitty's skin. Within a month of the surgery, I learned to administer these fluids to the old doll, once every two weeks or so. This step in her care should not have been necessary for months (or even years) down the road. Oh wait, I forgot to mention that more blood tests were recommended when a slight heart murmur was detected during one of the post near-death experience examinations. This most likely would have led to adding heart and/or blood pressure medication to this little creature's now weekly fluid administration, by needle under her skin, and the resultant anxiety (for us both, actually).

As best as I can recall the events during this blur, it was at this juncture that I decided to take my girls to a different vet, one reputed to use a more holistic approach to pet care and health, and to consider the wellbeing of the pet parents in the process. When Miss Kitty and I visited this new vet, we were at a point at which Miss Kitty was running away from me every time I tried to pick her up for a snuggle, because she was afraid I was approaching her with the dreaded needle to administer her fluids. Now let me emphasize here that I am not a medically trained person, and sometimes I made mistakes while poking her with this needle. On a few occasions I went too deep, drawing blood before I detected we had a problem. On a few other occasions, I poked the needle right through so that the fluid was flying into the air instead of under her skin. Miss Kitty was not at all happy about this process, which always took two people to complete. Given I lived on my own with my girls, this meant I had to either wait to "shoot up" my old doll until my sweetie-pie was visiting, or I had to ask the boy next door to help me inflict pain on my Siamese princess.

The good news is that the new vet's approach much more closely matched mine, than did the "by the book" approach of the other vet. However, I was soon to learn that even this vet seemed to want to keep in business the manufacturers of testing products and kitty meds. Somehow, each visit (and there were several), seemed to involve testing one of Miss K's bodily fluids, followed by antibiotics in the form of shots and then take-home liquid antibiotics, something else Miss Kitty simply hated to ingest. What happened to care and compassion that involved listening to the pet parent? What happened to honoring the pet's right to a peaceful existence and a good quality of life? Are testing and medication the only important pieces in current veterinary medical practice?

Menopause or Lunacy

The real bad news was that Miss Kitty then started to experience recurring bladder infections, apparently the result of her kidney problem. While the first infection cleared up nicely as a result of testing and the use of medications, within three months she experienced another infection. This time, however, she did not react well to more testing and medication. Her bladder infection persisted and her skin became extremely hot and itchy, and her general health continued to decline. So what did the vet say? Yup, you got it—more testing and medication. Where was the consideration for an old doll kitty who was having trouble negotiating small climbs that, in the past, she made without any thought or effort. Where was the care and compassion for her dignity? Was no one, other than me, her kitty mom, concerned about the distress through which we were putting this kind and gentle creature? Apparently not.

As a result of the "let's test and medicate" approach to kitty care, this kitty mom, afflicted with menopause-mush-mind, was left to determine to what extent she would allow her little girl to be poked and prodded, with the continual hope that she would experience a miraculous, albeit temporary, recovery and spring back to her former kitty-self. And why, when the writing seemed to be on the wall, was this decision so very difficult for me to make, when in the past I'd put my pets out of their misery at least somewhat more decisively. Or is this one of those memories which the mind alters as the years go by? Well, perhaps. But most certainly, my current age and stage of life were affecting my ability to make decisions about this sweet and loving pussy cat.

Was my lack of decisiveness caused by my ability to relate to Miss Kitty's age-related disorders? Did I understand all too well the negative impact of the aging body on the everyday patterns of life? When I looked at this beautiful, elderly cat, one minute I was clear that I must take steps to allow her old, unwell body to rest while her beautiful spirit flew free. In the next moment, with another look at her, I asked myself how I could so easily decide to take such drastic measures when she was simply getting old. Ah, but wait! She wasn't simply getting old. She had a very serious disorder that was causing these other conditions, meaning that no matter how many tests the vet performed and no matter how much medication he administered in order to clear up these ongoing problems, she would not ever be well again. Ah, finally I made my decision, which had been almost impossible because we were in a vicious circle. By allowing the testing and medication cycle to continue, I was really giving the old doll only a brief reprieve from the inevitable. Each time we tackled a specific small problem, I gave myself false hope that lasted for a few months, at best, until the next problem showed itself, calling for more testing and more medication.

I asked myself, if I were in Miss K's shoes (or should I say "paws"), would I want to simply exist on this poor-health roller coaster, so far from where I once was as a healthy creature, so full of life? I knew my answer to this question. I'd want to get off the roller coaster and make a dignified exit from my deteriorating body. So in this muddle called menopause-mush-mind, I had to grasp these moments of clarity and set Miss Kitty free. Yes, I simply had to do it for this very good friend of mine!

At that moment, I resolved to make the call the next day to the vets who make house calls, so the old doll could die with dignity in her own home. Then, Stinky Monkey and I would take her to my sweetie-pie's country home and bury her in an elevated place of beauty and serenity, where we'd allow her spirit to fly free, while her tired, old body welcomed a long overdue sleep.

Jottings

I'll Never Look Like *THAT!*

The physical changes and challenges
faced by women-of-a-certain-age

Don't Call Me Ma'am

The smashing of my left clavicle couldn't have come at a worse time. Come to think of it, quite likely, there is no good time to smash one's collar bone, or any other bone for that matter, but doing so at the age of 14, as opposed to 40, would have made for much faster mending. It was September 11th, just three days short of one month past my 40th birthday. While out for a quick bike ride, before settling in to paint my living room, I slammed my road bike down on its side on a paved park path, and in the process, smashed my left clavicle. Nope. No half way for me! I managed to break—no splinter, really—the bone in two places, ending up with a free-floating bit, about three-quarters of an inch long. When said bit floated, did it ever hurt! So at a key time in my life, when continuing my fitness regimen was rather important, I'd made it pretty much impossible to keep in good shape. I had to stay flat on my back, both to avoid excruciating pain and to have the bone heal in the least contorted way.

In very late January 1997, I decided it was time to head back to the weight room at Wilfrid Laurier University. I picked a time of day that was not overly busy, and set to work lifting light weights. In fact, I'd picked my timing so well that for a while a fresh-faced, lovely young man and I were the only people in the weight room, and while I sat resting in between sets, I amused myself by watching him work out. Or perhaps I was gazing off into space, thinking about my quick fall from a pretty darn good level of fitness. All right, I will confess that I just might have been feeling a tad sorry for myself, but I sure didn't expect what I heard next. Suddenly the lovely young man was approaching the bench on which I sat, obviously about to ask me a question. When it came, I was totally and completely unprepared, and I felt a knife plunge into my heart. Oh so innocently he asked, "Excuse me, ma'am. Are you finished with these weights?" And as I looked up in disbelief, there he was, smiling broadly and pointing to a particular pair of weights much too heavy for me to be using given my poor condition.

He continued to look and smile at me as I took a deep breath and answered, "Actually, I wasn't using them, so go ahead."

"Thanks, ma'am", he answered; swept up the weights with very little effort, and positioned himself at a station somewhat behind and to the side of me, where I could watch him as I looked forward and into the mirror.

Yes, it was true that just a few days previously, I had frightened myself as I looked into the bathroom mirror. Most certainly, the stress of pain had rendered my face much older looking than it had been just four and a half months earlier. Surely I hadn't sunk to "ma'am" status, had I? Woe was me! Suddenly I felt ancient and wondered what the hell had possessed me to choose a university weight room for my re-entry into weight training. Why had I picked a venue where most of the users were far younger than was I? The pain of it all. Wasn't it just a year or two earlier that the fresh-faced young men looked at me with intrigue and perhaps even wonder (at least in my world), knowing I definitely was older than they, but noting that I was in amazing shape. And now, I'd sunk to being seen as a "ma'am"—a fate worse than death. I finished my next set of repetitions and we were listening to the tunes and getting into the rhythm. I decided to deliver a set of weights back to the rack located near the one who had accused me of "ma'am-hood". As casually and lightly as I could, I thanked him for asking me if I was using the weights before taking them, because lots of guys didn't extend that courtesy. He nodded and said, "Hey, no problem."

"But, would you mind doing me a favor in the future?" I continued.

Not sure what was coming next, he looked a bit pensive and replied, "What's the favor?"

"Just don't call me ma'am, okay?" Then with a somewhat puzzled look, followed by a grin that told me he'd caught on to my meaning, he looked down, a bit embarrassed, and nodded.

As I settled onto another bench and set about lifting my newly chosen weights with much more authority, I pondered this change of status from intriguing somewhat-older-woman to "ma'am". I didn't much like it, and headed back into a thought pattern of puzzlement and disappointment. Could it really be happening that these sweet young things were seeing me as a woman so much older than they were? Isn't that what "ma'am" indicated? Sometime during my journey to feeling sorry for myself, I realized that two more fresh-faced young men had joined the first, and they were spying the set of weights with which I'd just finished. It seemed, if I heard correctly, that the first young man was telling one of the others, "I think she's finished with them ... just go and ask her. But, don't call her ma'am."

"What?", asked the second young man.

"Just don't call her ma'am."

"Okay", the other replied with a shrug, and headed in my direction. "Excuse me, are you still using these weights?"

As he pointed to the weights I was no longer using, I looked up at him and said, "Go ahead, I'm finished with them."

"Okay, thanks," he responded.

And then, just before he turned to walk away I added, "Oh, by the way, thanks for not calling me ma'am." Obviously I'd projected my voice enough for the others to hear, and we all had a good laugh, they somewhat embarrassed that their conversation had been overheard. I used the opportunity to explain to these lovely, young creatures that while they, undoubtedly, were attempting to be polite by using the term "ma'am" to address me, in fact, they were wounding me deeply. Seeing the puzzled looks on their faces, I continued to explain that I (and most other women) associated the term "ma'am" with much older women, and hoped that they didn't see me as their grandma, at least not quite yet. You can only imagine my relief when they all agreed, without hesitation, that I'd not yet reached granny status. Phew! At least I had a few more years left in me before they would equate me with the rocking chair set! Ma'am status was bad enough; but granny status would be a fate worse than death.

Always Wear a Pretty Camisole

Perhaps you've always been in the habit of wearing pretty undergarments, sometimes choosing camisoles and sometimes pretty brassieres or lacy things of that ilk. However, now in your menopausal years more than ever, the particular style of such garments is most important. "Why?" Did I hear you ask "Why?" I'm sure I did, and I don't blame you, so will launch immediately into my explanation.

Well, you see, assuming you are not in the habit of putting your naked breasts on public display, you must, at this point in your life, choose an undergarment for your upper body that covers well the bits you don't want to exhibit, just in case your outer garments must be shed in a moment of extreme hot flashing. Extreme hot flashes can cause the menopausal woman to suffer feelings of heat and suffocation so extreme that she must strip down, as close to naked as possible on her upper body, no matter where or when said hot flashing occurs. More often than not, this stripping down takes place without any thought as to her location or circumstance. All she knows is that if she doesn't find immediate relief

Menopause or Lunacy

from these extreme conditions, she will expire. So off must come the clothing that covers the upper half of her body. If a turtleneck garment is worn for some crazy reason, this dramatic stripping is all the more urgent. Let me explain further by way of example.

During a recent trip back from Seattle, Washington where a group of friends and I attended the Seattle Yacht Club's Opening Day—well, opening week, more or less—I was clothed in sailing gear to ward off the damp and chill the day offered. We had been travelling at 9 knots on a cloudy and sometimes drizzly afternoon and into the evening. Once into our moorage, we celebrated the good trip with a beverage or two in the cockpit of the sailboat, and then decided we'd best proceed to find a spot for dinner, given the evening was marching on. So without a moment's hesitation, up we got and were off on our mission. With some batting of eyelashes and such, we managed to find a lovely spot for our dinner, and proceeded to order, eat, talk, laugh, and imbibe another beverage or two. We are sailors, after all!

Others noted that the temperature was rather toasty in the restaurant, a fact perhaps exacerbated because the seven of us were cozied into one booth, so we were a tad crowded and with limited air movement. Intent on my extremely delicious bowl of Dungeness crab chowder, I failed to take these comments in the precautionary manner that would have been wise, for me in particular. All of a sudden, I stopped eating my tasty treat and realized that I was past the point of no return in my extreme hot flashing. Suddenly, it was imperative that I feel cool air on my upper body—a matter of particular urgency because I was wearing a turtleneck and a fleece vest. With my partner, Philippe, (who had introduced me to this wonderful world of carrying-on while on sailboats with other carriers-on) at one side of me, and our lovely male skipper on the other, I began the wiggling and jiggling necessary to get myself out of my vest. Then I pulled my turtleneck away from my neck and attempted to fan air onto my neck and chest using my hand. But alas, I was too far gone. Checking quickly with my free hand to ensure that I was wearing a suitable undergarment that closely enough resembled a strappy summer top, I kept wiggling and jiggling until I was out of my turtleneck, too.

There I sat, happily feeling air on my skin as I fanned myself, with everyone looking at me. My sweetie-pie, smiling at me, enquired, "Well, do you feel better now?"

I acknowledged that I did, adding, "Good thing I followed my rule for menopausal women to always wear a pretty camisole, or I'd be either in big trouble or a very popular woman right now!" They all acknowledged that had I been sitting at the table with them in a brassiere or with my bare boobies proudly displayed, they'd not have been upset, but I might have caused a stir in the restaurant and caused us all to be kicked out, thereby missing our dinner. And it would never do for a crew of hungry sailors to go to bed without our dinners and perhaps an additional drink, or two!

A Sleeping Disorder called Menopause

Quite often I feel I would give anything for a good night's sleep. Listening to my partner cry on my shoulder because he didn't sleep through the night, every once in a blue moon, I ask myself what the hell happened to my sleeping patterns "When did they change?" and "Will they ever return to 'normal'?" Or is this now normal and must I get used to feeling tired for the rest of my life?

While I'm tempted to blame my sleeping disorder totally on menopause, I must confess that that's not quite the case. I think I can blame the early stages of this disorder on a former partner who had a sleeping disorder he didn't want to investigate beyond a certain point, even though it kept me awake for the majority of nights of the entire three years we was together. Now why was it, I wonder, that I didn't awaken him and tell him to sleep elsewhere and instead always felt I was the one who had to leave our bed and locate myself somewhere quiet? Had I awakened him and told him to remove himself, I'll bet he would have been far more interested in further exploring his own sleeping disorder, thereby alleviating mine! Ah, good old hindsight!

Further on that point of respecting my partner's need to sleep more than my own, I realized it also was the time when my self-esteem took a huge nose dive, leading to, as I recall, my need to look toward my partner for my happiness. At that time, I attributed my dwindling fondness of myself to having burned out from my decade-long, once exhilarating job, and not having found a good replacement for that labor of love. I also attributed it to me not returning to my status as fitness addict after having broken my collarbone and having had to take it easy to allow my body to heal itself. You see, not returning to my former, all-encompassing quest for the rock-hard god-bod led to my body shape changing to a more human form associated with a 42-year-old woman who doesn't live in the gym, tossing about weights and ogling young boys. So when I looked in the mirror I no longer saw this rock-hard shape to which I'd grown accustomed—the same rock-hard shape for which I was admired by men and women alike, for being so fit "for my age".

Although I had never allowed myself to be financially stable, it was also during this period that my spiral into near financial ruin picked up huge momentum, with me attempting to buy true happiness by surrounding myself with neat stuff that I really liked, and which garnered me much attention and many compliments. Leos, after all, live for just this type of attention, and by buying lots of neat stuff and receiving those compliments from others, I could avoid the fact that I wasn't giving myself any compliments, couldn't I? But how much spending would it take to elevate those external voices to the decibel level needed to drown out my own negative comments about myself?

I find it very interesting that the spiral into low self-esteem and totally irresponsible financial management, described above, mirrors what's been happening to me since I've realized I'm menopausal! If I've been knowingly menopausal for about 3 years now, could it be that I was menopausal 3 or 4 years before that? Or, can it be that I was severely perimenopausal and that the condition caused me to choose that particular partner at that particular time, with that choice leading to all the events that followed?

Oh, my, I think I've hit on something here! In fact, although my sleeping disorder started even before I knew myself to be menopausal, it still can be attributed to this *maniacal* time of life called menopause. Stick with me now, and I'll explain why.

Back in 1998, for no one identifiable reason, I became disenchanted with my life, on a wholesale level. This disenchantment caused me to make decisions that led to self-doubt and low self-esteem. These choices included: starting a new relationship when I'd vowed to stay single for a while; leaving my job and moving to a new city; giving up my pride-and joy-truck, but not paying off as much of the loan as was possible, leading to increased financial concerns; and not returning to fitness endeavors, not even on a less fanatical level, once my collar bone had healed. Although life together was less than wonderful, I decided to follow my relatively new partner, and move clear across the country, and put myself into an even more intensely uncertain situation.

I think it is fair to say that during all these changes, made in an attempt to grasp the happiness that was eluding me, sleep also eluded me (most often because of worry). And I continued to add to my woes with my ongoing spending in pursuit of satisfaction and contentment. Then, my partner and I called it quits, a move that brought with it much sadness, even though it was the right decision. Then, much to my surprise, I met the man who seemed to be the love of my life—one Philippe! Even then, I kept spending money. Then the job that seemed wonderful derailed and I found myself in the midst of more uncertainty and, low and behold, in the throes of full-blown menopause, complete with hot flashes that kept me awake for a period of time each and every night.

Jeezy peezy, talk about your vicious circle. Obvious, even to me, was that I must find a way to break out of this cycle. Not at all obvious to me at that time was that I was entering menopause, a *condition* that I couldn't fix, and it was about to take me for the roller coaster ride of my life.

From Zero to Full Time Menstruation, and Back Again

It was my first trip of major proportions (well, if you can call three weeks major proportions, that is—but, to me it most certainly was, given that, so far, the good sailor and I had spent only weekends on the boat). And what a stroke of luck! You see, I wasn't menstruating! I hadn't been menstruating for a few months, and I showed no signs of starting again—no bloating, no full and tender breasts, no PMS sadness, etc. Of course, I packed plenty of tampons, just in case, because with having already missed several periods, I had every confidence that once I did start again, I'd need lots of *feminine protection.*

During the first few days of our trip, although I was wide-eyed with excitement and attempting to drink in all that this journey had to offer me, I was always on the lookout for signs that my dreaded periods were returning. But after that first week, I forgot all about such things. What a blast to not have to worry about the mess and discomfort of menstruating when I was living most of my days in bathing suits or in no clothing at all! This joy was all the greater given the rules and regulations that apply to boat toilets (or heads, as they are called). Let me explain, for those of you who have not had the pleasure of boating. Anything that enters the bowl of the head must be of a size or texture that can fit through a very tiny valve that mixes it with water and mashes it up. Then, under certain circumstances, the new mixture is sent through a very small hose and then a "through-hull fitting"—an opening that allows for this material to exit the boat through the ship's hull, while not letting any of the sea water back into the boat. So on a boat, one learns to use as little tissue as possible, and avoids sending a tampon down through this intricate system of ridding us of our waste materials. Therefore, they must be wrapped up in tissue and placed in the garbage; and, depending where you are boating, this garbage might have to stay on the boat for a week or more. So, as you can imagine, not menstruating while holidaying on a boat is a good thing, to say the least.

Well, I'm happy to report that my luck held and I did not have to deal with a period during that first holiday on the sailboat. As I recall, I did not have to deal with the joys of menstruating until sometime in October—when the floodgates opened. Yes, I went from no menstruation to lots of menstruation, including heavy periods (heavier than I'd ever experienced) and, in between my periods, spotting almost constantly. Along with the bleeding came menstrual migraines and extremely painful cramping. In short, I was paying, in spades, for my four or five months of no menstruation. It was in late November or early December when a nurse, with whom I worked, gave me proper heck for staying at work when I was bleeding so heavily that I was having accidents, even while I was using the most heavy-duty tampons you can buy and large pads (which I was calling feminine diapers). When I did not leave the office immediately upon her strong suggestion that I go home and lay down, she put in front of me the name and phone number of a gynecologist she recommended and demanded that I call immediately for an emergency appointment. By this time, I was frightened, and did just that, and within a few days, I went in to see this specialist. Then, of course, I was into the hospital for several tests to see what was happening in my girl parts, and to test my hormone levels. As a result of these tests, the good doctor was able to tell me that my hormone levels were such that I was well into menopause (something my girlfriend had told me several months earlier). He said that I had a significant thickening of the lining in my uterus, and that I had a cyst on my left ovary that he suspected wasn't a problem, but wanted to check more closely. Suddenly I had a date with this thorough gynecologist, at the end of January at a local hospital for a diagnostic hysteroscopy and, most likely, for a D&C.

While I awaited my date with the good doctor, all my difficult symptoms continued, including the continual spotting. All the while, my sweet sailor man

Menopause or Lunacy

was amazingly supportive about the situation. First, and foremost, I thank the goddesses (and Aphrodite in particular) that he was not freaked out about intimate relations with a menstruating partner. Otherwise, I'd have had to cope with having no sex at all for months— not at all a happy prospect for me or for anyone who knows me, given I become quite cranky when I don't get my good lovin'. And of course, not a happy prospect for my wonderful partner, either. Secondly, Philippe brought humor to this difficult time for me on a number of occasions, including one time that was particularly heartening. One evening close to Christmas I arrived at his digs to find that he'd just finished changing the bed so it was all fresh and clean for us during that weekend. Feeling completely disheartened that I still had no respite from continual menstruation, I dropped my bag to the bedroom floor and said, "Oh, Sweetie-Pie, why did you change the sheets? After all, I'm only going to get them all messy again."

Without a moment's hesitation, said Sweetie-Pie answered, "Well, you'll notice the sheets are red!" Well, I laughed and gave him a huge hug, because at least I didn't have to deal with being shunned by the man I loved because of my state of messiness. Yes, that's exactly how I felt—not dirty, per se, but, most certainly, messy.

At the time of my diagnostic hysteroscopy, which was a surgical day procedure, Philippe also showed his support, even though he was away (at a hockey tournament trip with friends, where I was to have joined him, but couldn't because of my date with the doctor). He arranged to have his mother pick me up and take me to the hospital, and for the elder of his two sons to pick me up and take me home. How sweet! As it turned out, how fun to see the looks on the faces of the other patients and the nurses, when in strode this very handsome younger man, and in a Coast Guard uniform, to boot, to give me a hug, and to take me home. What a hoot! I could see in their eyes that they were both surprised and, for the most part, supportive. In giving me those nods of approval, or perhaps admiration, they indicated that they appreciated that I'd landed myself such a strapping, young buck, who was sensitive enough to fetch me from the hospital. And even though I felt rather foggy and weak, I took his arm and grinned ear-to-ear as my escort and I left all those ladies to think whatever they chose to think. My guess is that they were grinning for some time after we left, and my hope is that my knight in shining armor brightened their day!

Well, as the good doctor predicted, I suffered two or three more heavy periods, albeit with lessening degrees of discomfort from headaches and cramps. And then, it was over. Well, I didn't know it then that it was over, but many years later, I look back to see that that was the end of my menstruation. As far as I'm concerned, that momentous event came not a moment too soon. Some women celebrate their menses, whereas I have fought it my whole life through. I could never figure out why, as a girl, I had to suffer each and every month of my life, when the boys had to do no such thing. I suppose, as well, that I resented the whole damn thing even more because I was not interested in becoming pregnant. So the only joy I experienced from getting a period was the assurance that I had not conceived that month. And because I was on the birth control pill for so many years of my life, I seldom had any doubt that my period would arrive. To me, therefore, getting rid of my periods, once and for all, was a cause for celebration, big time!

Looking back at it all, and talking with other women who experienced circumstances similar to mine, I have developed this theory. Our periods become even more problematic than usual just before they cease, so that, just in case a woman were to feel sad about passing beyond that stage of her life, she is bloody (pun intended) happy to get rid of that monthly happening and move on to a free and happy life sans periods. Besides, one can only hand wash one's messy undies and outer clothing for so long before becoming totally and completely exasperated, and the garments becoming permanently stained. Oh yes, and I'd be remiss here if I did not mention larger stained items, such as bedding right down to the mattress, and chairs of many varieties.

Donna Faye Randall

Come to think of it, I still can think of absolutely no good reason to celebrate the menses, except that it is an indication of no pregnancy—a very good thing when one does not want to be in the family way.

Hot Flashes—Yes? No? Can't Remember?

Sometime along the way into this journey called menopause, I started to develop a fever during my periods. How interesting, I thought. I'd never yet experienced fever during my menstruation. I'm not quite sure how many periods passed before I realized that perhaps it wasn't fever, but the start of hot flashes. I do recall that the realization hit hard, and gave me much cause to ponder my stage of life. I then set the entire matter aside and didn't think about hot flashes again, until my second summer aboard our boat, *Euphoria*.

Let me see, where was I in my process of menopause? Oh, it's already such a blur. You see, part of the self-defense mechanism provided to us, with this phase of our lives, is that our memories fail us to such an extent that we begin to forget about the chaos caused by menopause. If my rather pathetic memory serves me at all well, I'd already gone through my diagnostic hysteroscopy and accompanying D&C, and was several months into my latest phase of not menstruating—a significant improvement over menstruating day in and day out, and a real boost for my sex life. By then, Philippe's 30-foot sailing sloop, *Euphoria*, had become our nest at sea. I looked forward to spending three weeks with my man en route to, and in and around, Desolation Sound, that breathtakingly beautiful area of British Columbia where the ocean water temperature invites you to jump off the bow of the boat and to swim often, with or without a bathing suit.

My two favorite places on *Euphoria* are the cockpit and the V-berth. Anyone who sails will know why! (For those of you who do not sail, here is the answer: sunning, reading, socializing, and enjoying a quiet morning coffee and a bit of chocolate all take place in the cockpit. Blissful sleep after a busy day at sea, or at anchor, takes place in the V-berth. Perhaps most importantly, good lovin' is made in both locations!) But now, both special spots were to become sites of discomfort for me. That trip brought with it beautiful and hot weather; but anticipating some less desirable weather, we'd decided on bringing our regular-weight duvet, as opposed to the lighter, summer-weight one. As a result, we both awoke on occasion through the night because we were too warm. But my awakenings were of a different nature than I'd experienced before—they were desperate. I flailed in an attempt to avoid suffocating, with the only chance I had of cooling off being to shed my covers, starting with flinging my one leg out from under the sheet and duvet. I felt as though I was clawing my way

Menopause or Lunacy

out of a hole in the ground. But not long after escaping from the bedclothes, I was awakened again, this time because I felt cold, as my sweat-drenched body was exposed to the cool night air.

About two weeks into the trip, after a particularly chaotic night for me, the good Philippe made mention of my rather disruptive sleep and of the rather alarming heat radiating from my body. I wondered if I was fighting a flu bug, or whether my elevated consumption of alcoholic beverages (imbibed, of course, because I did not want to shatter the reputation of the drunken sailor) was leading to me doing battle with said spirits throughout the night, to rid my body of them (which I learned later was a contributing factor). Within a day of that conversation, in the cockpit while nude sunbathing, I experienced one of my suffocating bursts of heat. Suddenly and finally, I figured it out. These were the dreaded hot flashes of menopause, and they were no damn fun! Why had I been so daft about my hot flashes, given I knew I was past the peri-menopausal phase and well into menopause proper? I think this lack of association happened because I had been using natural-source progesterone cream for six or seven months, a concoction that I thought would help alleviate this particular aggravation of menopause, as it was alleviating the major emotional upheavals associated with *The Change*. But apparently, my cream was not performing that particular trick, and now I all too fully understood the power of the hot flash. Oh lucky me! Oh lucky Philippe! While his multiple reminders to me to use my cream had kept me out of the depths of despair during our vacation, we now were bathed in my sweat throughout the night. How were we to know? What was I to do now?

Well, given we had no alternate choice of bedding for the remainder of our first long boat vacation together, we pretty much had to tough it out together. I can tell you that I became extremely familiar with the port side of the v-berth, with me scrunching as far over and against it as I could, in my attempt to stay cool and keep away from my bunkmate. The heat factor became absolutely unbearable when our bodies were entwined. But this strategy led to its own problems for me, given *Euphoria* has a shelf running along both sides of her v-berth, about a foot from sleeping level. Every time I started to hot flash and flung my leg out the port side of the v-berth in a desperate attempt to find cool air, I'd slam my knee into the underside of the shelf, square on the top of my kneecap. By the end of the vacation, therefore, I sported a rather small but black, purple, and yellow bruise on that knee, and experienced significant tenderness there. And well into the winter of that following year, after we'd not slept on the boat for many months, that bruised kneecap remained visible and tender. (Having just looked at my knee as I write this scenario two and one half years after that fateful summer, I still see evidence of the bruise, although the tenderness finally is gone.)

Something I didn't know or even suspect then, but that I know all too well now, is that these hot flashes were to get far more frequent and far more impactful on my life, before they'd get better. Little did I know that I'd have to learn to make major adjustments to keep from sweating, or should I say "frying", myself into oblivion. In fact, over the next many years, I would struggle with finding the right combination of bedding in order to accommodate my many sleeping scenarios: sleeping with my kitties only, sleeping with Philippe only—both at his digs and aboard *Euphoria*—and sleeping with Philippe and my kitties. I would also struggle with making the choice of pajamas versus nightgowns versus sleeping in the buff, depending upon the sleeping conditions and upon my bedmate or mates, and upon the location of my attempt to sleep.

Through it all, there was severe sleep deprivation that adversely affected my entire life, extreme sadness that sleeping with Philippe sometimes had become an unpleasant experience for me, and agonizing frustration that nothing I tried seemed to help. And there was even a new hairdo created as a result of these nocturnal emissions of the female variety. Yes, the experience became hair-raising, indeed—and my hair had to be raised, in the style of Pebbles of *Flintstones* fame, a style that I am not convinced suited me well, but there it was, each and every night!

I'm inclined to deduce that, during those killer hot flashes, I sweated out and fried most of my brain cells. You see, it was not until a good five years after that fateful summer, during a sizzling hot one, that I clued in to remove the duvet from its cover and use just the cover, in order to sleep much more comfortably, Sheesh!

Did I Happen to Mention the Change in Body Shape?

As someone who believes that all clouds can have a silver lining, I've been trying, desperately, to find one in this menopausal cloud—well, aside from the obvious one, that is. Okay, the obvious one—other than not menstruating anymore—is quite obvious to anyone who knew me previously, and it was so succinctly summed up by my baby brother, David, as only a baby brother can do.

In the autumn of 2004, my little bro and his family, and my mother, moved to Vancouver Island from Ontario, from a rural area outside Cambridge, to be exact. But I digress—again. Upon Philippe's and my arrival for a visit one day, David exclaimed (when I was wearing a low cut fitness top), "Hi, Fayzie. Hey, you have breasts!" Asked when I got those, I explained that I grew them, just for Philippe, who grinned quite proudly, as I stood tall and stuck out my chest. You see, when I was a little girl, my older brothers used to call me "Boobless" (which of course I was, given I was a little girl!). My father used to comment that he'd laugh if one day I grew breasts so large that they entered the room several seconds before I did, so that my brothers would have to eat their words. While I was always grateful for my father's support, I'm rather happy his wish hasn't come true, because I'd hate to have to wear a bra at all times. Besides, not much sense in Dad's wish coming true now, given he's not here to see it happen. Oops, it seems that digression has happened, but this time without it surrounding Philippe. So back to the present and to that silver lining about which I was speaking—or rather, writing.

Yes, I was rather proud to have grown breasts that were large enough to produce cleavage, yet still firm enough so that I couldn't hold a pencil under them, between the boobies and my rib cage, when I was sitting or standing tall. However, said silver lining tarnished just a tad, at least in my eyes, given that the newly fuller boobies were accompanied by a generally fuller body, with way too much fullness happening in the area of the hips, tummy, bottom, and thighs—a plight most likely all too familiar to many of you. This added weight, and a shift of much of it to, or below, my waste, continued to bother me, especially as we entered boating and bathing suit season. One day, when Philippe and I were dressing for an evening gathering at the yacht club, or some such thing, he caught me standing in front of the mirror scowling at my reflection. When he hugged me from behind and cupped my boobies, he asked me, "Why the frown?"

I expressed my displeasure that my fuller chest had to come at the cost of much more Donna Faye down below. "The problem is", I explained, "if I lose weight and work out like a mad thing to return to my former svelte self, then my larger breasts will disappear along with my larger hips, tummy, thighs, and bottom."

Without hesitation, Philippe furrowed his brow, as if wondering what was the issue, and answered, "You just keep on feeding those boobies, and don't worry about the rest. You look great."

So I took the man at his word and continued to enjoy larger meals and more sweets than I had in previous years, while failing to increase my fitness activities to any measurable extent. Therefore, several months later, the chest was even fuller, but so were those other areas further down my body, and I was growing more and more concerned. So I started to cut back on my intake of excess food and returned to eating foods that suit me best. And back from the boat and into my non-summer-vacation routine, I started walking and cycling more. While I did notice a bit of a difference, at least in feeling less full, most certainly no miracles occurred. After much chiding of myself, I realized that in all likelihood I wouldn't ever return to my former shape, for two reasons. The first reason is that menopause simply tends to change the shape of our bodies while it adds a bit of extra fat. As I understand it, this extra fat helps us through the menopause phase, by helping us retain estrogens in our bodies, or some such thing. Honest, this isn't just something I made up as an excuse to keep feeding those boobies! The second reason I'll not be the rock-hard goddess I was in the past is that I really don't want to return to being that woman driven by exercise and terrified about having anything on my body that wiggles or jiggles. Of course, with the lack of desire to be that hard-bodied woman comes a lack of motivation to spend the ten to fifteen hours a week doing fitness-related activities. In the past, if I didn't do it, I would freak out. Back in those days, I truly thought that if I didn't maintain my rather exhausting fitness regimen I'd go to hell in a hand basket within days of missing just one workout. Ugh! I'm simply not interested in being that obsessed, or even driven, anymore. Hey, perhaps another silver lining of menopause is a re-ordering of priorities!

Okay, so why don't I finally get back to that silver lining thing, about which I've been writing? I have managed to find one, aside from not menstruating and growing those nice, full breasts. Are you ready? Well, in my quest to cull unnecessary stuff from my life, I work on my clothes closets. I find it so much easier to give away clothing that no longer fits me at all, as opposed to pieces that still fit me, even sort of. Believe me; such items number all too many, these days. If I really like the item, I'm tempted to keep it until I get back into better shape. But when I try it on again and see that it would take a loss of about three inches from my hips to make the garment fit, I assess what kind of workout schedule I would have to undertake. Then, begrudgingly, I place the piece onto the pile to go to the local organization that supports women leaving abusive relationships. As I begin to feel the pang of loss—of both the garment and my former body—I console myself that, not only is it a good thing to unclutter my life and enhance someone else's by donating this clothing, but also that my extra layer of body fat will help me through this very challenging, albeit sometimes humorous stage of my life.

I almost forgot to mention that, to my way of thinking, this culling also allows me to justify visiting my favorite consignment shop to see what Emmy has waiting to enhance this new, full me! And of course, I also remind myself that Philippe and I like my softer and fuller shape. Apparently, others do too, including my baby brother. Hey, let's see what happens when next I see my older brothers. Then I'll be sure to wear something that accentuates my newfound cleavage, and see if they notice. Surely they must do, given all their past comments about me being boobless and looking like their little brother.

Yikes! I just got up and passed a mirror. Am I sure that these full breasts and the accompanying estrogen-storing fat are worth this larger midsection? Ugh! Sometimes I still can't decide, fully and completely, if those boobies are, in fact, a silver lining of menopause.

Lotions, Potions, Serums, and a Good Deodorant

Back in the *olden days,* I was low maintenance, using the same soap and lotion for my face as for the rest of my body. In those days, the morning ablutions were of a reasonable length, so that I could get out of the house within 45 minutes of hopping out of bed, with a wee walk of my wee puppies (my beloved pets of the time) included in the process. Then, about the time I entered pre-menopause, my ablutions started to become longer when I started thinking that just this one new item would make all the difference…or, more likely, that this whole new line of products would do the trick. What trick, you ask? (Yes, I definitely heard you asking, now didn't I? And I will answer, but you will have to be just a bit patient.)

Anyway, with the addition of this and that to my morning routine, the departure time following my leap out of bed was delayed to the point that I had to plan for at least one hour of preparation time on a good day. On a bad one, the puppies and I would suffer, with their walkies being truncated, or completely eliminated from the routine.

Suddenly, when next I packed to go somewhere, even for just one night, I was amazed (and horrified) that I needed quite a large case for my toiletries, and the packing process took much longer than it had in the past. Then came 9/11, that fateful day when everything in the world of flying on commercial airlines changed, and we now had to be separated from our toiletries, rather than taking them in our carry-on luggage! The horror! The horror! Now we were forced to take the risk that they might get lost and not arrive at our destination when we did, and then what? What happened if we arrived in a country where we couldn't purchase the same line of products? And what if we were vacationing in the sun? Would our skin go into absolute ruin without this skin care regimen? What were we to do? Our vacation would be shot and our lives would be in ruin, don't you know.

We hit a slippery slope as we encounter major changes in the way we look and feel, and we stop enjoying the look of the person in the mirror. We fall into the trap of believing the marketers and our friends (other women who no longer enjoy the person looking back at them from the mirror). We believe that we can trick (yes, here's the trick of which I spoke earlier) ourselves into believing that we can buy back our former looks. I found it horrifying to realize that the success or failure of my life had been reduced to whether or not my toiletries arrived with me when I travelled. And that I resented the increased airport security precautions now in effect (even though they just might save lives) because I might not look, or feel that I looked, closer to my former self. Yikes! Okay, okay! So people are starving in this world, and perhaps even in the country where I have chosen to vacation. But we can't help that, and especially in the middle of this skin care product crisis, right? Oh, the horror of that kind of thinking—especially by me!

As if this change in my feeling of self worth wasn't bad enough, within a few years of it—a time I now realize to be my fall into the depths of the despair called menopause—I started to stink, in various regions of my body, and the hunt for an effective deodorant was on! I found this task particularly difficult, given I was trying to go natural with *all* my products. Now, let me stop here and explain the extent to which I had started to stink, because I can imagine that you all want to know this detail—in an up close and personal way. One clear (but still polite) example I can give you is that I remember being at a party where the music was too loud and one had to stand quite close to another partygoer to be able to converse. In the midst of one of these situations, while talking to a particularly handsome man (no, not Philippe, as these were the days before I went west, still a youngish woman not yet thinking about menopause) I detected a waft of unpleasant underarm odor, and recall thinking, with disgust, "Why would someone come to such an event smelling so unfresh?" Then, as the handsome man and I sat on a sofa to talk some more, and I raised my arm to lean my elbow on the back of said sofa and face the one-so-easy-on-the-eyes, I realized with much anxiety that the stinky person was me! While quite sure I was blushing with embarrassment, I removed my arm from the back of the couch, with as much grace as I could muster given the situation, and our conversation continued. But oddly enough, the man in question never did return my phone calls following our meeting, and who could blame him?

Eventually, having given up going natural, at least for this stinky phase of my life, I did find a good deodorant ... Avon's deodorant for men, if you can believe it. I'd always thought that I was a woman with more than the usual amount of testosterone, but who would have thought so at this time of my life? In fact, it was the almost never stinky Philippe who introduced me to this product, which I would use when staying at his digs. Low and behold, it worked! That was good news, although it broke my promise to myself to switch to all natural products, one that I was able to keep on another front.

The next product-hunting phase took me to birch bark oil, said to be effective in the fight against cellulite. I'd always been convinced that women got cellulite only if they didn't take care of themselves, even though I'd had a wee patch for much of my life. So when the patch grew, and a photo of me in a bathing suit during our first summer in Desolation Sound revealed beyond any doubt that I now had to worry about this condition, I hunted down and generously began to apply birch bark oil. (The wonderful Philippe took the photo and didn't ditch me when he saw my ugly body in the viewfinder.)

I have used the oil for many years, during which time my cellulite has not gone away but has not become horrible. I don't really know if it works, but am absolutely panicked by the thought of stopping its use, in case it does work and I would watch my skin deteriorate before realizing I must start using it again—and would I be able to reverse the damage I'd done by engaging in this experiment? So what if this stuff is rather costly? What horror might I cause by going off it only to find out I need it and that I need to spend the money on it.

Jeezy peezy! Will this expensive quest to return to look similar to my former self ever end? Perhaps not, I think, as I am shopping for more of the same and newer products. Perhaps what will happen is that I will realize that I never will return to being the same person I was before menopause, but I just might become accepting of, and even happy with, this new version of me. I can only hope that as my body settles into a new balance of hormones, the stinking and fussing will dissipate, and I can, and will, stop searching out new products.

Going Off HRT—Easy Does it!

When Hormone Replacement Therapy (HRT) was first introduced to the Western world, it, like the pill, was touted as a miracle for women. On the positive side, its creation and marketing at last offered women acknowledgement that menopause often proved to be a difficult time of life, and that physiological reasons exist for those difficulties. In other words, through marketing HRT, the pharmaceutical world admitted that women experiencing a trying menopause were not simply being hysterical. As a result, hordes of formerly hysterical women hungrily turned to HRT for relief of their extremely difficult menopausal symptoms, and found a magical relief.

Leaping ahead many years into the early 2000s, shock and horror rocked the world of the menopausal woman as research studies drew a clear link between HRT and breast cancer. I still puzzle, however, that the same link has not been drawn between the birth control pill and breast cancer, and surmise that this potato simply is too hot for the pharmaceutical world to handle. Time will tell. In my opinion, and as was the case with the introduction of the birth control pill, HRT was released onto the market without having been adequately tested, with women serving as the guinea pigs for this magic potion. Both hormone-altering medications were touted as being a perfect fit in a world in the throes of women's liberation and helped women avoid having to deal with their biological selves, while competing with men in their work worlds, and while attempting to be super women who could do it all.

All too suddenly, in mid-2002, the world crumbled for the multitudes of women on HRT or, like me, those starting to consider the merits of using HRT, with the hope of avoiding the agonies often associated with menopause. For me, the research findings prompted me to avoid the lure of the, by now, traditional HRT potions, opting to work with my body during this rite of passage, enlisting the help of wise women who'd already been there, and using natural source and herbal remedies. Huh! Easier said than done, but doable, particularly for the woman who has convinced herself that turning to natural products—lotions and potions, vitamins, and food, included—was the way to go in this world of chemicals and preservatives. However, for the women firmly dependent on the traditional HRT formulas, the news was more debilitating. Basically, they were hooked on this formula of synthetic hormones that allowed them to deny their menopause and to function without having to deal with its annoying symptoms. Without a doubt, I'd have been there, too, had my menopause started earlier than it did.

Many women and their doctors reacted out of fear and immediately stopped taking HRT. Suddenly they fast-tracked themselves into the menopause they had been avoiding, and suffered the simultaneous onset of all menopause symptoms, without allowing their bodies time to react to one symptom before moving along to the next. For a whole host of these women, the shock to their bodies, emotions, and lifestyles simply was too much to handle, and they returned to their former drug of choice.

Now, some women recognize (sometimes with the help of their doctors) that they need to taper off their use of these powerful preparations, and they are meeting with varying degrees of success in doing so. As I understand the situation, we know now that the previously used hormone replacement therapies deny the body its natural process of going through menopause, so it will have to go through that process once we stop taking HRT. The only way to avoid menopausal symptoms indefinitely is to stay on HRT until we die. In addition, with the link drawn between HRT and breast cancer, the HRT option seems far less appealing than it once did. My own rule of thumb, at this point in my life, is that any fix that requires me to artificially alter my body for the rest of my life is not a fix at all. In fact, it is the denial of a natural process, and almost always leads to no good.

Recently I had the opportunity to meet with a woman in her late 70s who was trained as a nurse and who had just spent a year of her life in a very troubling state of health. Once we'd established that we could converse on a more familiar level, she confided in me that her year of health problems was directly related to the hormone imbalance in her body caused by years of taking artificial hormones, followed by gradually stopping that addiction. Yes, she used the word "addiction" to describe her dependency on HRT, and strongly held that women are addicted to HRT and suffer terrible withdrawal symptoms when they try to break that dependency.

She asserted that in her case, this hormone imbalance led to severe arthritis symptoms, to the extent that she had difficulty getting out of bed in the morning, and had trouble walking, lifting, and using her hands for basic purposes such as washing herself, cooking, cleaning her home, and lifting her grandchildren. However, once she asked for and received testing for arthritis, she learned that she didn't have it at all, but that her hormone imbalance was causing these symptoms. So, with the help a good doctor who understands the power of hormones and the value of vitamin, mineral, and herbal therapies, she is overcoming her false arthritis and slowly is returning to close to normal functioning. But, she must be extremely diligent in taking exactly the prescribed amount of these treatments every day, in order to help her body heal. Looking to her nursing training, she commented to me, "We have had no idea of the power of hormones in our bodies, so we have tampered with them with abandon and now we are paying the price."

During her description of her year of extreme discomfort, my thoughts turned to the chaos of mind and body I had been experiencing for the past several years, and continued to experience with varying degrees of disruption to my life. My thoughts also turn to my mother, who was on HRT for years and then gradually stopped depending on the product, only to experience the joys of menopause at the age of 76. More recently, she told me about her shock at the rapid onset of arthritis pain. At that point she could hardly make her bed or, horror of horrors, lift her very young grandson, for whom she helped care on a regular basis, and who was making a huge difference to her life at a time of much change and adjustment. Perhaps my mother didn't have arthritis at all! Perhaps she could have found a natural way of easing her pain and improving her life.

As my visit closed with this wonderful and wise woman, whom I had only just met and with whom I had shared tales of menopausal trauma, I thanked her for her insights and wished her well on her healing journey. Then I headed home to phone my mother and share with her this newly acquired knowledge. With Mom being a very stubborn woman—er, I mean to say a very strong-willed woman—I knew I would have to revisit this topic many times with her before she'd take any form or action. Mind you, that little boy in her life and the horror of no longer being able to lift him might just be the catalyst she needs to seek help, as opposed to continuing to assume that she *simply* was arthritic and must live with that situation. To my surprise, my mother, with the help of her female doctor, did take gradual action, with her symptoms of arthritis diminishing dramatically. As a result, Mom was able to resume numerous activities with little or no pain, with her later years being active and fulfilling.

Herein lie the benefits of women speaking out and sharing stories of aging and change with one another.

It's Unanimous about Menopause, Boating, and (Not) Sleeping!

On many boats, including *Euphoria*, the master bedroom, so to speak, is the V-berth. Almost always, the inhabitants place their heads at the wider end of this space, measuring just a tad larger than a queen-sized bed, and the pointy end (for the feet) normally measures about six inches wide. As you can imagine (or already know from experience, perhaps), sharing such a bunk with another person, especially one bigger and taller than yourself, can be somewhat tricky, at the best of times.

Given that one's menopausal years are not necessarily considered the best of times, this sleeping arrangement can go from tricky to pretty much impossible, as I've explained in another scenario in this book, entitled "Hot Flashes—Yes? No? Can't Remember?" (If you've not already read said scenario, you might want to do so to learn of these trials and tribulations, complete with the tale of the multi-year bruise on my knee cap.) Wow! I've just realized that I've employed the technique of digression without mention of Philippe! Well, at least until now, having just used his name!

Okay, now where were we? Oh yes, I was about to share with you the gist of a happy-hour conversation among three menopausal, or post-menopausal, women held in the cockpit, (usually located at the blunt end of a boat, known as the stern) and outside in the fresh air. One of the women started to tell of her state of sleep deprivation, in response to a comment made about the glorious hot weather we were experiencing on our vacations. The initiator of the conversation had just spent three weeks in northern waters, where she was chilly most of the time. In response, the sleep-deprived menopausal woman (not me, for a change) launched into a tirade about her strategy to try to get away from her male partner and bunk mate, as she experienced hot flashes and night sweats. From the ensuing conversation, here's what we learned about our three male partners (yes, including my otherwise lovely Philippe), their sleeping habits in the V-berth, and our strategies to cope at this challenging time of our lives.

In a nutshell, they are bunk hogs. Because of their height, they feel it is their privilege to sleep right down the middle of the V-berth. Now don't get me wrong. They don't plan to take up this significant amount of space in the bunk. They just end up there at some point after they are asleep. This does not help us as menopausal women who desperately are trying to get as far away as possible from any other source of heat, while attempting to cope with our own overheating bodies. During these cockpit confessions, each of us told pretty much the same tale of woe, of pasting ourselves against the cool side of the V-berth, having decided on which side of our partners we would find the most space. We three also spoke of sometimes awakening to find ourselves stuffed into the top V on our side of the bunk. Our nighttime travels, in search of the best place to find space, took us there, and without us knowing that it had happened, we awoke, feeling rather achy and confined. Of course, once we had been fully awakened by this shortage of space, we all did give our partners nudges to send them over to their own side of the bunk, only to repeat the situation later on during the night.

We shared that each of our partners attempted to defend himself, usually using his extra height as his excuse. Perhaps the best response to their collective excuse came from the woman who originally launched the complaint and who blurted out, "Do you really think that your extra height gives you the right to use two thirds of the bunk space?" That quasi-rhetorical question pretty much shut down the conversation, and we turned our attention to other matters. I, for one, hoped that our open-air discussion, about this important, and obviously commonplace (and maybe even unanimous) problem, was overheard throughout the bay in which we were anchored. Perhaps it would launch similar conversations and cause other partners to think about their V-berth sleeping habits and maybe, just maybe, about altering them.

As for one male involved in the conversation, I am happy to report that my Philippe obviously took our comments to heart. Starting that night, and continuing into the rest of that trip (and I can only hope beyond), my caring partner pasted himself against his side of the V-berth at the beginning of the night, and stayed very much on his side of the bunk until morning. And, on the occasions when I've been sleeping somewhat curled up and then attempted to extend my legs down to the bottom "V" and brushed against his leg, he involuntarily (or apparently so) has moved his legs over to make room for mine. Oh, the power of not suffering in silence, and of discussing our menopausal (or other) woes openly and with a pinch of humor added for easier digestion!

Thank goodness for this seemingly minor victory, which has led to better sleeps and happier times for both Philippe and me. I can only hope that reading this scenario has helped, or will help, many other boating couples to enjoy the time in their V-berths more than they have been during menopausal meanderings at sea!

The Road Back to Fitness

With my body now in a shape I've always identified with older women, I was having a terrible time motivating myself to get out there and get back into good shape. Don't get me wrong here. I wasn't setting my goal too high by wanting to be back in my mid-thirties rock-hard shape. In fact, I didn't really even want to lose weight, and therefore lose my new-found, full boobies. I merely wanted to be more taut, feel stronger, and have more energy. Even this goal seemed to elude me. Because Philippe's son and daughter-in-law owned a few Curves franchises in California, about which they raved in terms of the results their clients achieved, I set aside certain biases, and joined a local franchise. Admitting that perhaps I'd reached what I then thought of as rock bottom for me, off I went, faithfully and dutifully three times each week, to engage in circuit training. Just when I'd get into the groove of a move, I'd have to change to the next station. However, the other clients were fun, as were the staff members, and the walk to and from the gym added to the workout and provided me with some enjoyment. But I never felt as though I had a really good burn and within about six months, I had to force myself to go.

I knew I was in really big trouble when, about ten months into my membership, I'd start out for my local Curves, but walk right by and to the beach, then up the shore line and around back home—a pretty good workout in itself. We had just returned from our three-week vacation on *Euphoria*, in Desolation Sound—complete with its swimming, hiking, dancing, and fun, in general. Quite simply, I could *not* force myself onto that horrifyingly boring circuit, the same thing day in and day out! While millions of women worldwide found their fitness quest fulfilled in Curves franchises, this situation was not for me. In so many ways, I enjoyed and admired the women who could stick with the Curves plan and reap the benefits, but I realized I was not one of those women. So what now? What was it that would capture the interest, and therefore earn the devotion, of this former fitness goddess?

I cast my mind back to a conversation with a friend in Desolation Sound, a woman about three years my senior and in very good shape. She biked to work almost every day—in her work clothes and on a hybrid bike. Well now, I worked not too far from my home and sometimes walked home from the office. But, given my difficulty getting up and ready in the morning, I could never spare the 40 minutes I needed to walk to work. However, I could spare the 20 minutes it would take to bike! Yes, that was it! I needed to buy that cruiser style bike I'd wanted for several years and start biking to and from work. You see, it seems that I always needed to make a purchase to start a new endeavor, and this was a perfect excuse to buy that lovely style of bicycle. After all, mountain bikes did not lend themselves to biking while wearing your work clothes. Yes, I could get fenders and higher handle bars for my mountain bike, but that crossbar simply wouldn't work.

A woman on a mission, I had my research completed and my new bike purchased within about two weeks. And bike to work I did, at least three times per week. Then the rainy season in Victoria was upon us, and I most certainly did not want to ride my pretty bike in the rain, now did I? So cycling fizzled, except on nice days, when I'd take long bike rides. But, that wasn't enough to get me in shape, and my decline into the depths of fitness despair continued rapidly—well, at an alarming rate, actually. More and more clothing stopped fitting me, and while I liked the breasts I'd grown, I wasn't at all fond of my larger thighs, nor my wrinkly legs and saddle bags. How had I become this frumpy, middle-aged woman? Most certainly, I knew that menopause was doing me no favors in terms of my body shape and weight gain. But that was no excuse to stay in such poor shape.

Then one day, as I sat in my office, a co-worker and friend passed by, said hello, and then returned, in backwards motion. "You'd do it with me!" she exclaimed.

"What would I do with you?" I asked, not wanting to say yes to anything unless I knew into what I was getting myself.

"You'd take belly dancing classes with me, wouldn't you?" my friend asked.

Immediately, I knew my time had come to become a belly dancer—for fun and fitness! "Yes! When? Where? Sign me up." I shouted with glee. "I can't believe your sense of timing." I added. "I'd love to take belly dancing classes with you!" So we registered for the next session, and were scheduled to become belly-dancing queens immediately after Christmas holidays. This time, I knew I'd found my niche.

Jottings

Finding Myself

The spiritual changes and challenges
encountered during *The Change*

Is it Possible to Forget This Stage?

So, after carefully listening to my excitement-filled account of this book that I was going to write, this book about menopause, with a humorous approach, Philippe asked me, "Now, don't you think you need to be further along in your menopause to be able to write about it? Don't you think it would be better to tell your story after you've been though the whole thing?"

Damn he asks good and thoughtful questions, I said to myself, hummed and hawed around a bit, and then said, "You know, Sweetie-Pie, that's a very good question, and I think I have two answers for it. Do you want to hear them?" Valuing our relationship, of course he said that, indeed, he did want to hear my answers. I then proceeded to explain that, first of all, I think you don't know when you are through menopause, any more than you know when you start menopause. Secondly, I think that the one major blessing of menopause is that you forget much of it, especially the really difficult stuff, once you haven't experienced it for a little while. So the best time for me to write about my menopausal experience, as a warning to others, is now, when I'm in the midst of this wretched journey.

After some moments of silence, the good sailor responded, "You know, that makes perfect sense! Do you think you'll really forget about all this crap you are going through?"

"Yes", I replied, explaining that I'd already lost some memory of the earliest of my intense menopausal experiences, and know that happened to several women I know, including my mother.

"Do you think I'll be able to forget about your menopausal experiences?" he asked with hope in his voice, hope I dashed immediately.

"Nope", I explained, "You don't get that privilege cuz you haven't had to endure these experiences."

"Like hell I haven't!" he argued.

Now, let me tell you about my mother as her menopause story relates to the blessing of forgetfulness. My mother had an interesting, and not particularly pleasant, menopause, especially prior to starting on Hormone Replacement Therapy (HRT), which was pretty darn new in those days. My mother had her fourth baby when she was eight days shy of 40 years old. Four years later, she was in a car crash resulting in neck and back injuries, accompanied by migraines, which she'd suffered most of her life. As was the thinking in those days, particularly when dealing with a woman who dared to speak out, the doctor prescribed my mother Valium and painkillers, which she stayed on for too many years, it seems to me. Looking back now, I think either the accident or the drugs jettisoned Mom into early menopause, because in the years that followed the crash, she suffered depression, refused to discipline her young child, lost all interest in cleaning the house, didn't have much energy, and seemed generally indifferent. I remember that we older children met and determined we would provide Mom and Dad with a good excuse to leave the house for the better part of a day and would then band together and do a major house cleaning for Mom. (You see, in our family Dad held no responsibility for, and apparently no interest in, anything even remotely domestic, so we were cleaning the house for Mom, not for Dad.) We presented this house cleaning as an act of kindness just cuz, to avoid hurting our mother's feelings.

Several times when I was a working as a sexuality educator, and then during menopause when carrying on about my menopausal experience, my mother made bold statements that she didn't suffer any menopausal symptoms. At first, I would bite my tongue and let her think that was the case. Finally, one day I took the risk of commenting that she must hold much different memories of that time than do I, because I seem to remember her menopause experience much differently than did she. During our discussion that followed, she commented that because she hadn't experiences hot flashes, she felt that she hadn't had a difficult time with menopause. It seems, you see, that she'd forgotten all the other ways in which her life was turned upside down, back then. Now, perhaps I'm off the mark and her behaviors were not menopause-related, but were, instead, the result of the car crash injuries and the resulting drug use. But since our conversation, Mom has made note that her periods stopped not long after those injuries. She also has noted that she'd forgotten much of that experience until we'd talked about it.

So, to my way of thinking (and as a result of this very scientific and extensive research), we just might be blessed with the forgetfulness of menopause, which allows us to disregard the intensity of our menopausal experiences, even if we don't forget the experiences fully and completely.

Belly Dance—an Answer is Found

From the first class, I loved belly dancing. We'd been lucky and found a teacher who valued belly dance as a form of expression that honors women—our physical structure and our inner selves. Yes, doing it well and performing might be what some of us would decide to do with our art form, but Sidona Moon enjoys teaching the women who take her classes for no reason other than making them feel good and more self-confident than they did before starting.

    I loved the way Sidona started and ended each class with yoga exercises. She made learning fun and told stories of how frustrated she was when she was first learning, and still is when she has trouble with a new move or dance choreographed by someone other than herself. Immediately, I got into the whole thing and purchased a jingling hip scarf from a woman who had been to Turkey and brought back some middle-eastern treasures. I also purchased zills (the things that belly dancers click with our fingers) and a set of videotapes to help me learn and practice at home. I looked forward to each class, and was sorry for the two-week break between my first and second beginner level sessions.

Part way through my second session of classes, Sidona Moon announced she was putting together a new dance troupe for Folk Fest in early July, and asked those who wanted to join the troupe to talk with her after class. Of course, I did just that! I was the only one in my beginners' class who did so. I became very excited at the prospect of putting together a costume and performing on stage. But more than that, through belly dance I was finding my way of being in my current body form, which was much changed from when I was hard-core into rugged physical fitness. Suddenly, I was appreciating and honoring my more curvaceous and softer body, including my hips and tummy. And when I headed to class or practiced at home, I felt confident in my middle-aged femininity!

At the end of my second eight-week beginner session, Sidona Moon asked me to stay on for the intermediate class and join the dancers who were to make up the dance troupe to perform at Folk Fest. Immediately, I enjoyed the women and enjoyed learning the choreography, and putting the steps I'd learned into action. We started to rehearse twice a week and meet for class once each week—and we started to create our costumes. Sidona Moon believes in encouraging us to express our individuality through our costume choices, giving us only a few guidelines: that we wear choli tops, circle skirts, straight skirts, a tunic, and head coverings, in various combinations, depending upon the origins of the dance number. She asked us to focus on the jewel colors—a guideline still offering much freedom. I have to say that I was amazed by the excitement and fulfillment I experienced in choosing my costume pieces, based on what felt right for me.

    Rehearsal after rehearsal, each troupe member arrived with new bits and pieces of our costumes, each brimming with pride and with all of us expressing our appreciation of the choices. Even though we all put together costumes of similar styles, the variation and the individuality expressed truly was amazing. And rehearsal after rehearsal, as we looked less at Sidona Moon's feet and more at our own, and stored the dance steps into our muscle memory, the dances took shape and we all began to blossom. After many hours of rehearsal and practice, we all knew the numbers well and didn't have to concentrate so hard on either "what comes next" or our feet. We began to envision our audiences and to smile for them, and at times even flirt with them. As we grew more confident within ourselves, we gelled as a troupe and showed still more support for one another. We were increasing our fitness levels so we could stay on our toes, lift our chests, use our stomach muscles for undulations, hip circles, and chest circles, all the while holding our heads high, smiling at our imaginary audience, and adding the sultry emphasis necessary for enchanting belly dance.

For me, the crowning glory came on the day of the performance. That morning we had breakfast at Sidona Moon's house, and applied our makeup and dressed in our costumes. Together, we walked, as a troupe, to Victoria's inner harbor to perform at Folk Fest. While we'd had a small audience for our dress rehearsal the evening before, we now had a *real* audience, complete with our own friends and family members. When I spotted, in the stands, my sweet sailor man, who had seen none of my belly dance moves, I shone and got the feel for the sexiness of our dances. And of course, I felt extremely proud and accomplished. Within six and a half months of taking my first class, I had become a performing belly dancer who truly had embraced the art form and knew the basics of this exotic dance. Of course, I knew I had lots more to learn, and looked forward to learning it all.

Yes, this art form, this fitness activity, this confidence builder, and this form of camaraderie were part of me, and I would keep working hard to become an accomplished dancer and performer, all the while enjoying my newer, fuller, and more feminine, middle-aged body.

As it turned out, a combination of activities has been most helpful for me in navigating my way through menopause, while maintaining a modicum of fitness. As I continued to maintain a focus on belly dance, I

Menopause or Lunacy

returned to Curves for several years, eventually giving that a rest and turning to NIA (a dance based body movement program) and Svaroopa Yoga. By talking with menopausal and post-menopausal women, I have determined that each one of us needs to find our own road to fitness, all the while attempting to enjoy ourselves as we try to keep our changing bodies happy and healthy.

The Woman I'm Becoming and the Electric Pink Shoes

I was no longer using my hormone replacement cream (ran out and, with my doctor now retired, simply hadn't replaced it). My hot flashes were annoying but not devastating and my mood swings were tolerable. My energy level was on the rise, and I was getting back into more fitness activities. I was even considering heading to the local recreation center for some serious fitness gigs...but not having done so yet, I was getting out on my bicycle more often. All was going well—and I was re-introduced to Converse shoes, and the fabulous store that sells them in downtown Victoria. Having fallen in love with the lime green models on the sweet feet of my nephew buddy, I simply had to get to that store and check out those shoes. To add fuel to the fire, my nephew's mother sent me the store's website link, and I was off into the world of Converse.

The very next day (after combing through the website), I found an excuse to head downtown and took a wee side trip to Baggins (as in Bilbo, perhaps?) Shoes. Well, I was so mesmerized that I wandered around the store for the better part of an hour, wanting one of everything! In fact, I loved so many of the shoes that I feared I'd have to leave the store without making a purchase...most unlike me! But just as I was about to leave, I spotted them. Bright pink with shiny silver undertones, almost like lame, they caught my eyes and wouldn't let them go. I never wear pink, but this was pink with attitude. And then there was the part that can be folded over to look kind of like baggy socks at the ankles, complete with the amazing patterns and colors—circles, triangles, stripes—in pink, yellow, green, teal, and blue. Wow! What was not to like? So I bought them, and merrily toddled my way back home, pink shoes safely tucked into my shopping bag.

That night (or really very early the next morning), I awakened because of a combo of hot flashes and having to tinkle. Then, as I attempted to return to sleep land, I was haunted by my purchase. Why had I chosen pink? I don't wear pink. I have nothing that will work with the shoes. Besides, wouldn't I look silly in them, having this time gone beyond that line of what a middle-aged woman should wear? Visions of my clothing pieces passed through my head as I attempted to match these items with my new shoes, and eventually I fell back to sleep.

In the morning, once I'd eaten, I took a good look at those pink shoes and started to comb through my closet and drawers. And ya know, I realized this pink was such a neat color that it would go with all kinds of colors, even with those that should clash. Then, of course, there are the other colors on the turned-down part that tie in with loads o' stuff. I set the shoes on the floor, sat at my computer, and began to work. As I turned toward the filing cabinet and the pink shoes caught my eye, the reality hit me: these are not pink shoes, but electric pink Converse, with funky tongues and flaps—and what in the world am I worried about?

In fact, at that moment, I understood that these shoes were perfect for me right here and right now, as they were my *coming through menopause, here I am liking the woman I'm becoming, being exactly who I am and who I want to be, look at me pink shoes with attitude.* Of course, they were here to stay!

Life's a Blast!

Although you might not have suspected a cry of glee from this author—this tired, often feeling old, menopausal woman—occasionally it happens. Some days are diamond, even for us, the tired, old crones. Or shall I say us, the tired, not-really-old, crones-in-training? Yes, I shall say that, indeed.

My day continues to be a treat, as I write with my lovely Miss Catianna, aka Stinky Monkey, at my side! Now, what has made me, this complaining menopausal maniac, so damn and disgustingly positive about life? Well, it seems I must admit that some days are diamond, whether in large ways or in rather small ways. To me, a day is diamond when my feelings of joy outnumber my feelings of frustration, sadness, desperation, and despair. I know the latter part of that statement sounds extremely desolate, and I don't mean to be dramatic, but, that's often the way I have felt since entering this phase of life. I won't elaborate ad nauseum, given I do so in many other segments of this book. Besides, this is a happy chapter, not a sad one. To illustrate what differentiates these diamond days from my far less happy (dare I say "gravelly") days, I invite you to please join me while I explore such a day from beginning to end. But wait, that's not quite so easy as it sounds, given my broken sleeps caused by my dreaded hot flashes— and they are all the more prevalent when my lovely, the sailor man, arrives to share my bed with me and Stinky Monkey. It makes it rather difficult to determine when my days begin and when they end.

Okay, so I'll start here, at 3:38am: I looked at my bedside clock, aware that I was awake and very, very warm. Since I was awake, I might just as well make the short trip to the bathroom to relieve my bladder pressure before returning to the blissful state of sleep until the alarm would sound at 6:25am. Having pitter-pattered to the bathroom and back, and having tried out several different positions sufficiently far away from both Philippe and the sweet kitty-cat to keep me from melting from the heat generated by my own body, I could feel that I was beginning that dreaded spiral into fussing too much and sleeping too little. However, by using the powers of diversion, such as petting the wee Stinky Monkey, and watching Philippe sleep, both while thinking of the positive aspects of my life, rather than the negative, I fell back into a deep enough sleep so as to be surprised to hear the alarm sound to begin the *productive* part of my day. I could feel the effects of sleep deprivation as the alarm sounded on my clock radio. Philippe had slept poorly too. We three were all too hot, and I made a mental note to change the duvet to the lighter weight one when the sailor man stayed with us, now that the nights were less chilly. Our combined heat led to poor sleeps for all (well, except maybe for Stinky, who seemed to sleep well under almost any circumstances, unless my leg flinging about, trying to locate cool air happened to flip her onto the floor.)

All too soon, however, Philippe was out of bed shaving and preparing to shower. He was off to Seattle and Portland to promote the Swiftsure International Yacht Race, and he needed to catch the floatplane on time, so he was up and at it. As I did most mornings, I used applying my eye drops as the excuse to luxuriate in bed for as long as possible. Before long, I was joining Philippe in the shower. Today was an exciting one for me too, as I was starting a new contract with an organization for which I hold much fondness; helping them raise more money was going to be a pleasant task, indeed.

Not long after Philippe left, I was ready to head out. My morning at the agency was an informative and pleasant one, and I liked the staff very much. I spent some time after my morning meeting choosing appropriate cushions for my home office chair, and buying a new halogen bulb for my home office lamp. Then off home to lunch with the Stinky Monkey before continuing my morning's work, which I packed up by about 6pm, fully intending to attend a forum on the right to die with dignity. Then, as I hastily ate my salad, I realized I had very little interest in scurrying off to said forum, given I knew my stance on the matter and really had little desire to discuss it at length.

Instead, I would write a snippet for my book, and would call my *other mother*, Maw, a very good friend from my Planned Parenthood days. Well, didn't we have a delightful conversation, interspersed with our craziness we call humor. During the conversation, I heard I had an incoming call, and decided to ignore it and allow the answering service to pick up. Once my call with Maw ended, I checked for my message and, sure enough, I'd missed a call from another Ontario friend with whom I'd left a message, who, in turn, left me an amusing message—almost better than having a voice-to-voice conversation with him. Not to worry, we'd talk later.

As I hung up the phone from retrieving Hugh's message, I scratched the kitty and exclaimed, "Stinky, life's a blast—a thoroughly delightful ride, if you choose to board the bus!" Suddenly I was filled with the wonder of the twists and turns of my life, and extremely thankful for the path I'd followed to date, and the splendid people I'd met along the way. Had I changed any piece of the puzzle, I'd have missed out on meeting someone or another very important to me, and that, Miss Stinky, would never do. They all are treasures, in one way or another, and through my association with them I am becoming a wise, old crone (or shall I say hag-a-training), and, most surprisingly, happily so. Yes, I've always wanted to be wise; but, no, I've not always relished the idea of being either old, or a crone, or hag. However, the truth is that one can't avoid getting old, unless one dies young (which some days along this journey has seemed like not such a bad idea). In spite of my earlier fears, and my failed efforts to remain young, and making a complete fool of myself in the process, I suddenly realized I was aging quite gracefully (well, except for the menopausal mania part), and with a good sense of humor to clear the path.

My friends, old and new, and old and young, offer me strength and guidance; and my loving man helps me feel sexier than I've ever felt, even when compared with those days when I was rock-hard and fit. Philippe knows just the right things to say and do to help me understand that accepting my femininity is a positive step for me as I learn that a new twist to my feminism is to celebrate the role of the crone, or hag, in our society. Damn it, I'm doing just that and having a blast! So, look out world!

The Hair's the Thing

For much of my life I've worn my hair very short, much like a male style but with a tad of pizzazz. I suppose it had a lot to do with bucking the norm. However, the ease of it certainly kept me heading to the salon for my haircuts, as did the fact that short hair suits me and is part of my identity.

I clearly recall one occasion, when I was heading to Ellicottville, New York, for a ski weekend with friends, and had stopped at the duty free store for a bottle of nice scotch for the weekend. As I stood looking at the choices before me, and therefore with my back to the other customers in the store, I heard a voice from behind me remark, "That has to be Donna Randall over there looking at that booze!" Now, even though I tended to drink a bit more booze in those days than I do now, I was confident that the fact I was looking at alcoholic beverages wasn't what lead this friend to recognize me at that shelf, but rather the fact that my hairstyle was distinctive enough to reveal my identity. And a quick question to my friend confirmed that the hair was the thing that caused him to notice and identify me so quickly and surely.

Most certainly, my short hairstyles suited my fitness activities of weight training, running, road cycling, and mountain biking. So I think I see my transition to long hair—at the time when I'd moved across the country, stopped most of my fitness endeavors, and (unbeknownst to me) started on my slippery slope into menopause—as a shift away from the me that I knew, admired, and respected. Come to think of it, as I've moved through my menopausal mania, I think it safe to say that my hair length and styles have shifted, first away from the former and stronger me, and now back closer to that former me, but in a new and improved version, or so I like to think!

As a chameleon, I tend to morph in and out of various incarnations as I move in and out of the various circumstances of life. Therefore, I am not particularly surprised that, while settling into life as a sunshine and sailor woman beyond the west coast, I decided to grow my locks so I could wear a ponytail through the opening at the back of my sailing hats, to keep said hats secured on my head while at sea. But perhaps most importantly, I recall feeling that a change in appearance would suit the life changes I'd recently embraced. So achieving long hair status became one of my goals.

At the outset of my journey into the world of long hair, I managed to connect with a hair stylist very near my place of employment, who knew how to cut curly hair, and seemed to understand the challenges in the process of growing one's hair, while attempting to keep it looking attractive during the process. And so JP became my stylist and hair trauma counsellor, and within three years I sported fairly long hair, and within five or six years, at the time of my 50th birthday, my locks were long, indeed. I had been through much of the menopausal experience but still had more to come.

Then, in 2008, I suffered a great shock when, one day, I called my stylist/hair trauma counsellor to book an appointment, and learned that JP had retired from the profession, but was told that someone else there could help. Well, someone did cut my hair, but really didn't help. I wasn't at all pleased with the result. Following tryouts with several different stylists, and after our summer aboard *Euphoria*, I went to a friend's stylist and decided to try something quite different for me, which was to have the back of my hair cut considerably shorter than the front (all the rage at that time), and so began the ramping up to the return to short hair. Then followed two more stylists, and various haircuts along the same lines, all of which I found lacking. Finally, in the autumn of 2009, having determined it was time to shed the longer hair and get back to being the real me, I located a wonderful stylist and took the leap—but not before conducting considerable internet research into various shorter curly hair styles.

When the day came, in consultation with Gerard, I opted for a short cut, but one not as short as my previous one-inch long hairs styles, to take advantage of the length of hair with which we had to work. Gerard was thrilled when I recommended an asymmetrical style. By the time we were finished, I was ecstatic about the new 'do, although I knew that my west coast blonde pony tail kind of guy might not be quite as thrilled as I. But c'est la vie ... the real Donna Faye Randall was back!

To my way of thinking, one of the first things we notice about a person is her or his face and head, and the hair really is the thing that is most noticeable. For many of us, when we feel good about our hair, we carry ourselves taller and in a more confident manner than when we don't like our hair cut, or when it needs a fresh cut. For me, this change back to short hair, but not the same style as in the past, has symbolized shedding much of the trauma of menopause that has oppressed me for a decade or longer. I feel great about the new 'do, and don't miss my long locks at all. Mind you, I do rather miss paying for only three visits per year to the stylist, rather than the six visits or more I have to make now to keep me looking striking, or as close to it as possible.

Patient Times to Come

Sometimes, when I'm not in the state of menopausal mania, I feel happy, patient, and at peace with myself and with my surroundings. During these moments, I catch a glimpse of my life post menopause, and I gain hope that this state will come to me sooner than later.

One summer not long ago, I learned, at long last, that Philippe likes to think that things are his idea, and then he takes to them very well, indeed. So I've learned to make subtle but clear suggestions (plant ideas, as it were), and then give him time to percolate and digest, and slowly turn these ideas around to being his. That summer, our long trip aboard *Euphoria* included one of these experiences, with a result very important to me. You see, on previous Desolation Sound holidays, I'd accompanied the good sailor northward and then returned by car, so that he could extend his holiday with friends able to stay out and play, and deliver the boat back home as the spirit moved him and the weather permitted. On this particular holiday, because I'd started my new business and had client commitments (and the truth be known, because I needed the money), I agreed to meet Philippe about five days into his trip, at Heriot Bay on Quadra Island. There we'd start a jaunt northward before heading back down into Desolation Sound to meet with friends and enjoy the warm water for swimming. Because I wasn't experiencing the trip up to Quadra, and because I'd not yet been included in a trip home, I very much wanted to head home with Philippe that year, and visit the little bays of which he spoke, and which I'd never seen. This feeling intensified as we said goodbye to two couples as they headed back down to Victoria, thereby completing their holidays as couples, in the manner in which I wanted to complete our holiday.

One night over dinner, I proposed the idea that, instead of carrying out an idea previously discussed, which saw me leaving on my birthday with a friend heading back home by car, that we leave together by boat a few days prior to that time, and head down the coast and across the strait together, arriving home by August 16th. This plan would allow us to celebrate my birthday on the way down the coast. I further reasoned that the summer was shaping up in a way that, if we stuck to his original plan, after I left, Philippe would have no buddies left up in Desolation Sound, so he'd have no play mates or travel companions. While he didn't reject the idea, he did make some noises about not wanting to cut short our time in Desolation Sound. I shrugged and commented that I thought this might be a good year for us to return together, especially since his buddies were all heading home early—being careful to keep the tone light and matter of fact. Well, it was two nights later, over dinner, that Philippe came up with the idea that we leave Desolation Sound on August 16th or 17th and make a quick trip home so that I could be back for my clients, just a few days later than planned. Tempted to leap at the idea, I pondered and then responded that I simply couldn't afford the extra days without working, and that whenever I got to do the trip home I wanted it to be a slower trip, allowing for time to visit his favorite anchorages. I proposed that the latest I could leave would be somewhere around August 11th, getting back home on the 16th. Again, the subject was dropped. Then, the next day, didn't that man o' mine have a new idea? Yes, indeed, he suggested that we leave Desolation Sound on the 11th or 12th of August, and he proceeded to offer up an itinerary for a trip that would see us visit his favorite haunts and have me back by August 16th. I listened with amazement that he honestly believed this idea was his, and then set to pondering the plan for some time, before agreeing that the idea was a good one—almost ideal, in fact.

Over the next few days I gave Philippe ample opportunities to change his mind and revise our plans (because I never want my free-spirited man to regard me as someone who forces him to do things he doesn't want to do), but he was keen on his new plan. So you see, without me having to become crazy and desperate, and raise a stink, or be sad, we settled on a plan almost exactly as I originally recommended and what I really wanted, because I was patient and waited for Philippe to determine a course of action that was his. (Oops! I sure hope he doesn't read this scenario, or he'll be on to me, and my new method—of patiently waiting him out, to end up with what I want—will have to be revised, just as I'm getting used to it. Yikes!)

I'm firmly convinced that my newfound patience comes from me starting to come through to the other side of menopause, a time during which almost every day involves panic, impatience, and complete frustration. Mind you, I acknowledge that women wiser than I realize much earlier in life that the way to encourage a man to see things from a woman's perspective is to plant the seeds and let them think they thought of the brilliant plan. But alas, me growing up with boys and always wanting to be like the boys, I didn't develop my feminine wiles until very late in life, and I sure am happy that finally, I understand.

The New, Period Free, and Mostly Happy ME!

My mother used to say that she was surprised by her age, and I used to think her very strange for her surprise. Now I understand her feelings of surprise and amazement, and fully agree with her explanation that we keep feeling like we've always felt about ourselves, but when we look in the mirror we see that we are inhabiting a much older body than our feelings tell us. From where has this body come, I ask myself, and what happened to my other, much younger body?

Interesting, isn't it, how our mothers grow smarter as we grow older? Indeed, my mom used to say some very silly things, but more and more now, many things she said I understand and relate to, with much more regularity than when I was in my thirties and younger. Hmmmm...

Also interesting that my mother was correct, yet again, when she said that all our experiences in life, although they seem horrific at the time, turn out to make us wiser, more confident, and less fretful than we were in our earlier years, even though we felt stronger and somewhat invincible back then. But what did we know... really?

One thing I know for sure now is that my mother and my girlfriends have been invaluable to me over all the years of my life, and continue to be so. I also know that I attract more and more magnificent women into my life as I mature and grow closer to being a wise, old crone—with each and every one of these women enriching my life, as I enrich their lives. For example, the following professionals in my life are wise women: my massage therapist, financial adviser, doctor, former belly dance instructor, most clients, all-time favorite consignment shop and specialty clothing store owners, yoga teachers, hair stylists, the two bankers who helped me through a crisis related to my mother's finances, and my business image and website consultant. What I would have done or continue to do without any one of them is beyond me. Why I ended up being in charge of my late mother's financial affairs is an even deeper question, and one far beyond the scope of this book.

So instead of that story, let's get right down to the heart of living a good life beyond menopause, which is, quite simply, cherishing the freedom of not menstruating! For me, the lack is the gain, and every time I hear younger women refer to having their periods, I think to myself "poor you". I think back, now about 8 years ago, to when I spoke with a colleague somewhat older than me. This woman had dragged herself into my office, plopped down onto my guest chair, and declared that she felt like crap. When I enquired about her ailment, she responded, "Oh it's my bloody period".

After I stopped laughing about her choice of words, I looked at her quizzically and exclaimed, "Surely you are not still menstruating!" Immediately realizing my incredible lack of tact, I expressed sympathy.

Now many years later, I almost can't remember menstruating. But whenever I am hand washing my pretty under garments, I marvel how long quality ones last, provided you don't put them in the washer, and how new they continue to look now that they don't wear the blood stains of unexpected periods, and especially the unpredictable and heavy ones of early peri-menopause. Long gone are the days of carrying around pads, tampons, and liners, or using them as a precautionary measure to ensure you don't end up in a puddle and attempt to hide the fact from everyone around you, even though you strongly suspect they know what's going on but are saying nothing out of kindness—or perhaps embarrassment. Gone are the days of ducking into the closest washroom, even if that means going into a corporate office (as I once did at the BC Transit Office), hoping beyond all hope that you will be greeted by a female receptionist who will recognize the look of panic on your face and direct you to the nearest washroom, whether or not it is intended for public use. Gone are the days of having to calculate, as best as possible, the dates of your future menstrual periods months in advance when booking a boating holiday, a holiday at an exotic seaside resort, or any holiday, come to think of it. Because a naughty time away just isn't the same when your uninvited period shows up. In fact, I clearly recall a close girlfriend of mine quietly sidling up to me at her wedding rehearsal, while wearing a beautiful creamy white dress, and whispering in my ear that she was in need of a tampon, or several. The excitement of it all had brought on her period about a week earlier than scheduled. And this wasn't a case of a young and inexperienced woman messing up, but rather a 30-something, second-time bride figuring it all out, only to have her body betray her.

To my way of thinking, the menopausal journey represents the last gasp of breath in our reproductive journey, with the menstrual cycle hanging on for dear life. Thinking of this battle between the two forces, I suppose we should not be surprised that it can be quite onerous, as the respective sides try to gain control, leaving the woman in question simply wanting it all to end. Okay, so if that is what menopause is like for some women, what's up with those who seem to breeze through the whole process? Well, my scientific description goes like this: I don't know. We only hope that we are one of the lucky ones who breeze through menopause, and ask those who experience very few issues to be kind and sympathetic to your less fortunate sisters!

Jottings

The Bottom Line?— *The Afterword*

So where are we at the end of it all? What's the bottom line here? Am I menopausal or crazy? Indeed, this was the all-encompassing question early in my menopausal journey.

Of course, the answer is obvious: *yes* to both prongs of this question! I have spent a long time experiencing both menopause and lunacy, with menopause causing, or at least exacerbating, said lunacy. So I can only hope that I have become at least somewhat less of a lunatic, having spent much time and energy working my way through this thing called menopause. But having made that statement, I must ask several questions:

- How does one know when one is completely through menopause?
- Does one remember how crazy one was during menopause, and therefore able to tell if one is any less of a lunatic once through this stage?

- Can those around us let us know if we are any less crazy after, than we were during, or indeed before, menopause?
- Does it matter if we remain complete lunatics or become lesser lunatics? Perhaps that's why older women own a license to be *eccentric*, the label given to women who wear odd outfits with the ability to pull them off because they really don't care what others think?
- Won't it be rather enjoyable to be regarded as *eccentric*? After all, many of us enjoyed lots of practice during our menopausal years at being very eccentric, so it would almost be a shame to become *normal* once again. Of course, that statement assumes that I was normal prior to menopause, and I'm sure I know a plethora of folk who would argue against that assumption.

Say, maybe I'll do something crazy like get a tattoo or some interesting pierces once I'm on the other side of menopause and am a crazy old crone! No, wait, I've already done that … twice with the tattoos and many times with the piercings. Or what about wearing a brush cut? Oh, I've done that, too. Oh, I've got it. I'll buy a Harley and become a motorcycle mamma. Yeah, that's it! Rats! Oops. I've done that, as well.

Ah, but here's the deal. Here's the beauty of having made it to the other side of menopause, be it difficult or relatively easy: we gain Crone Power. As wise, old crones, we often choose to stand up, clearly state our true feelings and beliefs, and fight for what we believe. When I think of the number of women-of-a-certain-age who have achieved great things for themselves and for the world at large, I feel proud to have reached this stage of my life. By Jove, I think I've got it! This vision of the next phase of my life works for me, perhaps because for my entire life I've tended toward activism for change. What's important, I think, is for each of us to find and do what fits our leanings and way of life.

So what do *you* think? Is there a bottom line to this menopause thing, or is this just another of life's experiences, when going with the flow is the ticket to survival? I'm thinking that in the school of "life is what you make it—celebrate it", perhaps *that* is the bottom line. And we know we are pretty much done with the worst of the menopause thing when we truly can celebrate it. As I write this Afterword, which really is a bunch of pondering and musing, I figure I'm at the point in this journey where I can, more often than not, celebrate my menopause.

Now what about you? Is your experience one of making your way through the murky minefield of menopausal mush-minded madness? Is it one of full-time or occasional lunacy? Are you having, or did you have, a relatively anxiety-free menopausal experience? Or are you not yet there, or are you just setting out on your own journey, and perhaps are hearing tales of horror from your mother, older sisters, aunts, or friends and colleagues? Maybe you are reading this book on behalf of a loved one and can relate this experience to her? Whatever the case, I hope you'll share your thoughts, feelings, experiences, fears, and hopes, for the benefit of our sisters.

Thank you for reading *Menopause or Lunacy...That is the Question*.

~ The end...and the beginning ~

Oh, Something More

Based on my experience, it is easy during the menopausal years to blame everything on menopause, in much the same way as we often, throughout our menstruating years, blame everything on PMS (Pre-Menstrual Syndrome). The major concern about falling into this trap is that we might go without tending to the symptoms of health conditions unrelated to menopause. Accordingly, I encourage regular visits to your health practitioners, as well as visits as indicated by changes in your body. Please remain vigilant, and true to your usual health monitoring practices, and respond accordingly. If you go out searching for books and other resources about menopause, you will have no difficulty finding many, and so I will pick only one book to mention. It often was recommended to me and I found it very helpful: *THE WISDOM OF MENOPUASE: Creating Physical and Emotional Health and Healing during the Change*, written by Christiane Northrup, M.D., author of *Women's Bodies, Women's Wisdom*.

Please visit me at menopauseorlunacy.com to check it out and join in the conversation, if you so desire. While you are there, feel free to follow the link and see what else I'm up to. Cheers!

Old Women (and Me)—A Poem

~ inspired by a conversation with my
younger bro, following a visit to the doctor
with our 81-year-old mother ~

Until recently,
    when I saw an old woman attempting to shuffle her
            way
      through a crowd of people, rushing to and fro,
        I'd pause and say to myself,
"One day, that will be my mother."

And then, not so long ago,
    I spent the day with my mother,
    helping her with her multiple stops for groceries,
    I became distracted;
    and when I looked up to see an old woman
    attempting to shuffle her way
    through a crowd of people, rushing to and fro,
    I paused and was startled to realize
    that the old woman I saw
was my mother!

Since that day,
    I have paused often, and thought,
    "If my own mother has grown to be an old woman,
then what of me?"

After all,
    when on a the bus and I look up
    to see an old woman attempting to negotiate
    the steps, her bags, and her bus pass, ticket, or money,
    I pause, then look down and up again,
    only to realize that one day,
    sooner than I care to think,
that woman will be me!

Donna Faye Randall

CPSIA information can be obtained at www.ICGtesting.com
Printed in the USA
LVOW11s0949130514

385462LV00001B/6/P